BE YOUR OWN BEST FRIEND

CHESSIE KING
BE YOUR OWN BEST FRIEND

Thorsons

Thorsons
An imprint of HarperCollins*Publishers*
1 London Bridge Street
London SE1 9GF

www.harpercollins.co.uk

First published by Thorsons 2020

10 9 8 7 6 5 4 3

Text © Chessie King 2020
Photography © Ruth Rose 2020
With the following exceptions: pages 13, 135, 183, 186, 189, 190 and 192
courtesy of the author
Illustrations © Saskia Robertson (Sassrobcreative.com) 2020
With the following exceptions: pages 32, 40, 76, 78, 113, 122, 162, 197, 207, 211, 214,
223, 232 and 224 © Shutterstock.com

Chessie King asserts the moral right to be identified as the author of this work

A catalogue record of this book is available from the British Library

ISBN 978-0-00-837739-7

Printed and bound by PNB Latvia

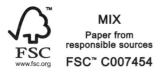

MIX
Paper from
responsible sources
FSC™ C007454

This book is produced from independently certified FSC™ paper
to ensure responsible forest management.

For more information visit: www.harpercollins.co.uk/green

CONTENTS

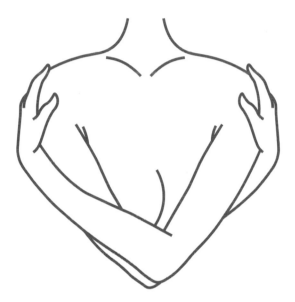

DEDICATION
This is for my Scrumma-mumma-doo-dah
This is for my Brontë Bee
This is for my best friends
This is for YOU, yes, you

Introduction

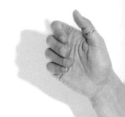

GIRLS. WOMEN. LADIES. ANGELS. GODDESSES. SISTERS. NON-BINARY READERS. (And to the guys who have bought this book, I see you … I know you want to see what it's all about.)

This book is all about the glorious, delightfully complex truths of **Femalehood** and becoming your own **best friend**. We're going to discover your true worth, big up your self-appreciation, find your inner cheerleader and celebrate **you** – zooming in, zooming out, while shaking it **all** about.

I believe there are four layers that make up you, me and the book you're holding.

★ Our insides: hormones, emotions, feelings and our juicy bits.
★ Our bods: boobies, body hair, periods, contraception, sex and all the things we didn't get taught at school.
★ Our solar support system: your community – the spine to your life – your family, the people you work with and your friends, your tribe, because there ain't no hood like sisterhood.
★ Our outer orbit: social media bollocks, people's views on what women 'should be' and connecting with strangers.

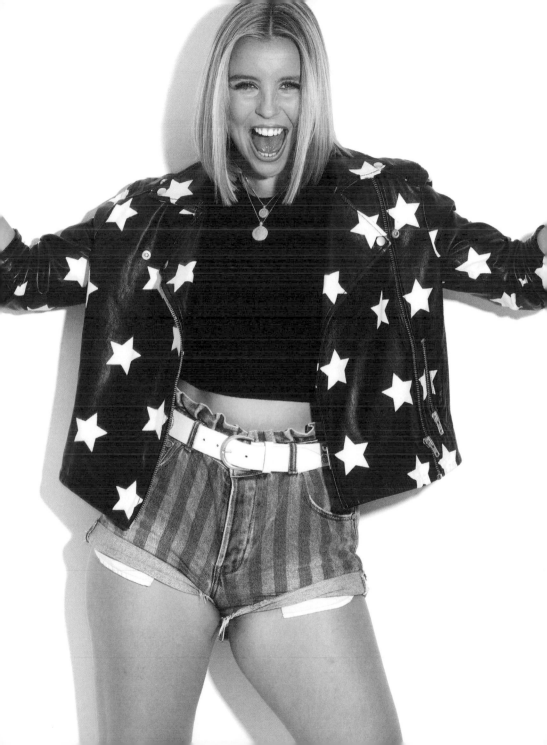

Every single one of us is navigating our way through life and sometimes, in this huge, gigantic world, you can feel like you're doing it **on. your. own.** It's a jungle out there, but I hope, while you read through, you'll be nodding your head like 'Yes, uh-huh, this is totally me – oh holy mother of Dorothy, I thought I was the only one. Phew. WOW. Okay, so if Chessie's been through this too, I've totally got it.'

I invite you to take a comfy seat in my brain, my world. I've poured love, honesty and memories into this baby. I've cried into my laptop, laughed at the stories I've unearthed in my history bank, and braved sharing unspoken pieces of my past. And heavens to Betsy, I have absolutely adored this whole never-written-a-book-before-what-am-I-doing thang!

My scrumma-mumma-doo-dah fired me out into the world on 23 June 1993, so I know I've not yet experienced **all** the bonkers things life can throw at us women. But I want to be dancing around in my underwear until I'm 100 – so I'm not even a third of my way through the game. I'm absolutely no expert, nor am I trying to 'fix' you. But I believe I don't need a PhD or a degree to want to help you or to share my life, my stories and my advice with you. I can promise you, this book is so much more than me telling you to sleep more, eat your veg and step up your step game … We're going to take back the power, we're going to turn surviving into thriving, we're going to become the CEOs of our busy brains.

We're all unique, we're all multi-dimensional, we're all phenomenal – however, the majority of us just don't **believe** in ourselves. Whether you feel like you've lost confidence, never found it or you're going through a shift, I'm here with you. In *Blue Peter*-style, *here's one I made earlier*: I've tried and tested the infinite list; exploring, discovering and unpeeling the layers of myself over the years. So, I thought it was about time I got it all down on paper … 240 pages' worth of paper.

You can be your own best friend
You can be your own cheerleader
You can be your own soulmate
You can be whatever you
want to be

I like to think of us all as scrummy, spongy cakes. We all started out the same, cooking in the womb. Then over the years, we've added in different ingredients, soaked up different experiences, to make us all even more delicious and **unique** ... But we've been decorated with heavy toppings like self-doubt, comparison, heartache, trauma, grief ... they're all baked into our lives and they could be weighing us down.

When **you're** ready, we'll work through your recipe and eat cake together. We'll **strengthen** your relationship with your bod, your brain, with all of the incredible humans that make up your tribe, and with women from all around the world.

If I could describe my Instagram in one word it would be '**honest**'. But unlike social media, this book has been a real safe space for me to take that to the next level. To help you, to share everything with you, **uncensored**. Helping, guiding, nurturing and supporting people is something I feel I was born to do. It's written in my DNA, embedded in me from my mumma, my mum's mumma (my nana), her mumma ... all my female ancestors have exuded love. I'm a big sister in real life (anyone who's the oldest will know what it feels like to be the 'trial run', the guinea pig) to Brontë and Henry, and I have always wanted to protect anyone younger than me. I've watched them both grow up from teeny tiny beans in our mumma's tummy, making their way through life, growing into their own individual personalities. I don't ever tell them **what** to do; I just guide – sharing with them my mistakes and what I've learnt. I celebrate their differences, encourage them to do **anything** they want and absolutely **adore** them.

This book is for **you**. Think of it as having a book-sized me with you at all times. I'm here with you on every single page. I want this book to be a constant reminder that you are abso-bloody-lutely extraordinary, so keep it close to you: in your handbag, on your bedside table, on your desk at work or under your pillow. Pick it up

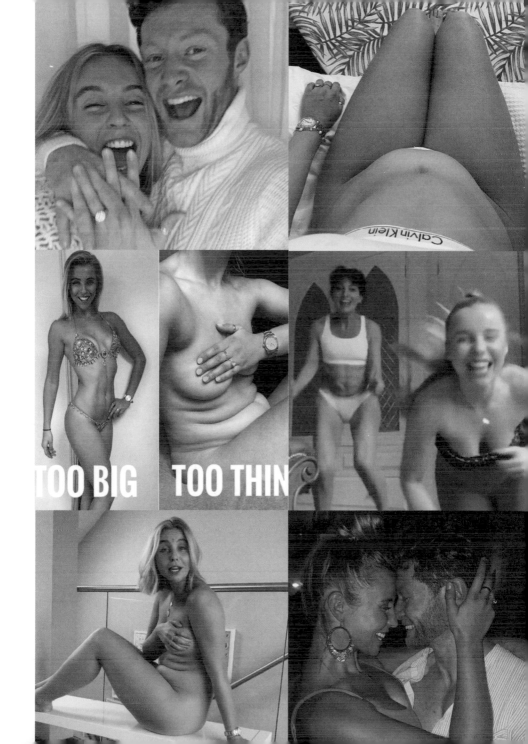

TOO BIG   TOO THIN

when you need a boost, and know that you can always come back to it in this wild, wild world.

There is absolutely no judgement here from the pages, the words, the book or me. I want you to feel like I'm reading every word out to you in real life (which, if you're listening to the audio book, I am!). I love scribbling, getting things down on paper, so I've added interactive parts to help you discover new ways to express how you're feeling ... so if **you** want to doodle, please do(odle!) ... or if you'd prefer, scribble everything down in a *Be Your Own Best Friend* notebook.

Put your hand on this page and take three of the deepest breaths you've taken all day. I've just done it with you. Are you ready to come on this roaring voyage with me? Are you ready to unleash that badass warrior inside of you? Shall we do this? **Yes, yes, yes, Chess. Let's go**.

SQUILLIONS of love,

Chessie x

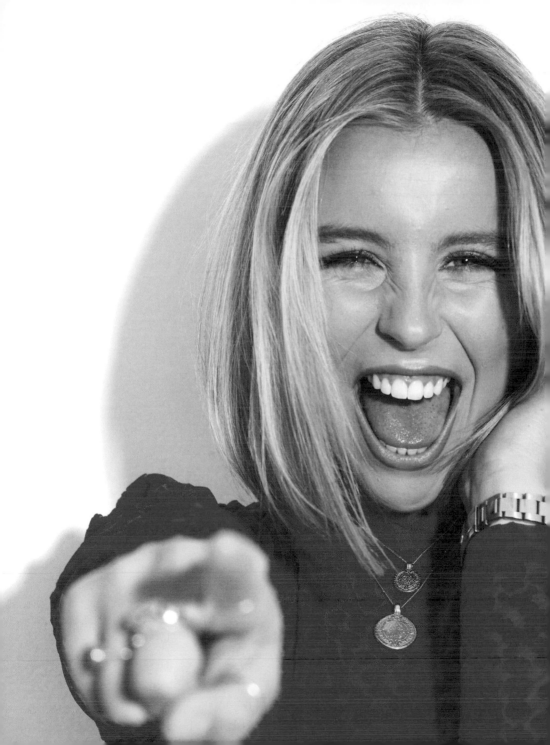

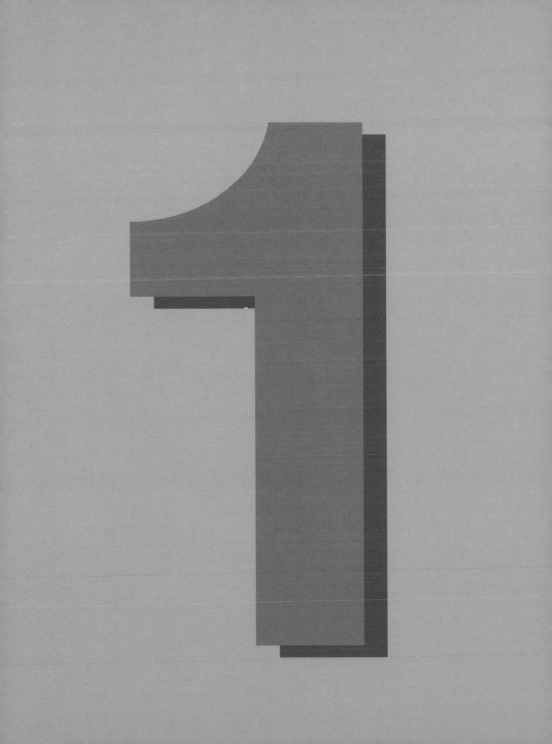

INSIDE US

REVEALING THE FEELINGS AND DEALING WITH THE HEALING

Inside us

Every woman is made up of what I like to call our 'juicy bits'. The bits we find once we strip back all the outside layers and delve deep into our centre – our core.

We've all heard, 'Oh don't worry, it's just all going on in my head' ... Wellllll that's because it **is**, but we need to talk about it. Our brain's function is to think – she's the powerhouse, she's the boss. Our juicy bits are our feelings, our emotions, our likes, our dislikes, our hormones, our thoughts and our unique personalities. Those sensations we feel have the power to dictate our days, our entire lives. Our feelings and emotions are the realest thing we have, they're unique to **us**. They're how we connect with ourselves and with people's souls, but they're invisible – so no one in the world really knows what's going on inside there. Not our partners, our sisters, our parents who've known us since day one, our friends – and sometimes not even **us**.

You know those people who don't yawn when you yawn, like they're immune to the infectious, contagious yawn? Well, I'm not one of those, I'm totally the opposite ... I'm extremely empathic. I can't walk past another human crying without wanting to make sure they're okay and have a good cry with them. As I've got older, my feelings have deepened, my emotions have developed, and my hormones ... well, I'm still trying to make friends with them.

My coping mechanism to deal with painful, harder, more complex feelings used to be to cram them out of sight in a

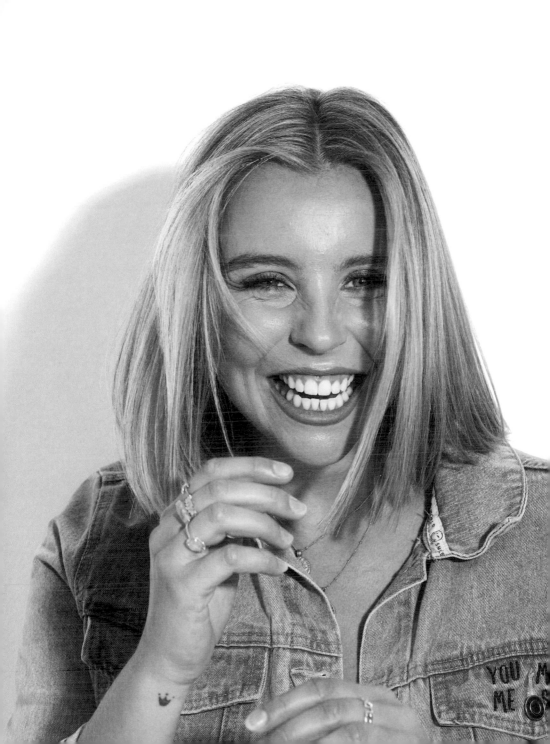

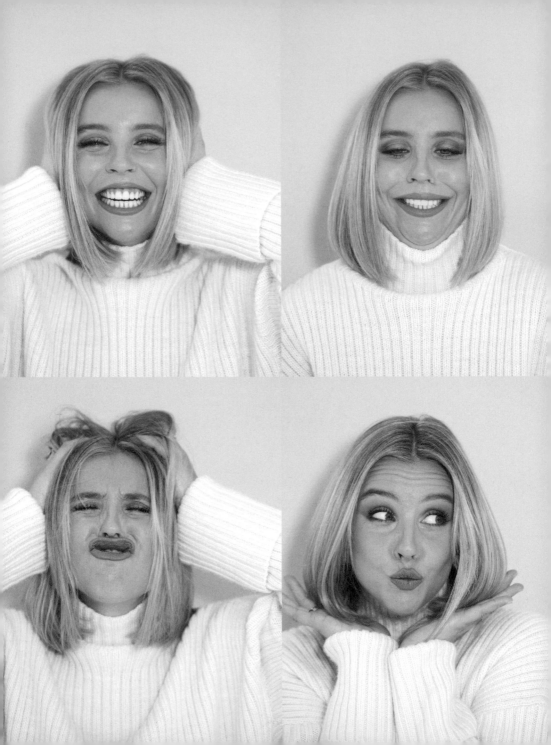

metaphorical box. But that ended in an exhausting emotional extravaganza whenever the box got too full and burst open. I thought the only emotion I was allowed to feel was happiness, that crying was a weakness and everything else was unnecessary. In my early twenties, I morphed into a robot – an empty, emotionless, 'I'm tough, I **got** this' kinda gal. I was presenting on a red carpet most evenings, working silly hours on top of that and giving up my spare time to surface-level relationships with absolutely no grit about them whatsoever ... plus I don't think drinking eight coffees a day to make up for the lack of food helped at all. I lost a chunk of myself while giving so much to my work, funding the coffee industry (with what probably added up to £20+ a day) and pouring energy into boys who covered up their cheating by saying they were dedicated to the 'polymonogamous life' (which I have absolutely nothing against ... when both parties are aware there's more than just you two involved – which I wasn't for 5 months!). Oh I definitely learnt a huuuuge amount from all of it – but it took suddenly losing my hearing and becoming partially deaf at 23 to realise I need to release these emotions when I feel them.

With the help of people talking about their mental health and sharing their own stories, I'm much more aware of my emotional self. I'm forever checking in and learning about what's going on inside me, understanding what I can do to harness a feeling or how to give myself a little bit of extra love when I need it.

SO THIS ISN'T ABOUT 'FIXING' YOUR EMOTIONS – I'M NOT BOB THE BUILDER. IT'S ABOUT:

★ Recognising them
★ Harnessing the power of the fiery ones
★ Helping out the more complex ones

And most importantly, if you thought you were the only one feeling 26 different emotions a second then hopefully, reading this, you'll start to see I'm feeling it, your best friends are feeling it, your cousins, your boss, your work colleagues … **we're all feeling it**.

In this section, we'll delve deep into our cores. We'll zoom in and uncover the layers that we've built up. I want to help you **peel** them back and hopefully get to know your most authentic self, your cake before all the toppings were added. We can learn to trust and accept our emotions – the good, the bad and the messy … they are a way of **celebrating** ourselves, **expressing** ourselves and **trusting** ourselves.

THIS IS YOUR DAILY REMINDER

YOU ARE NOT ALONE
YOU ARE SUPPORTED
YOU ARE IN CONTROL
YOU ARE STRONG
YOU ARE UNIQUE
YOU ARE LOVED

... NOW GO GET IT

Check in with yourself

How are you today? How are you really feeling? Trust the first thing that comes up with no judgement, just recognise it. Today might have mixed up a complicated cocktail of emotions – this is your time.

You're always asking how everyone else is but the more we get to know ourselves, the stronger our relationships with ourselves. Every day is an experiment – notice when you're feeling the happiest version of yourself. Remember who you were with, remember what you were doing, remember where you were. Get to know what makes your heart feel full.

BRAVE 28

PROUD 36

HONEST 42

CALM 50

SWAMPED 56

NOT GOOD
ENOUGH 62

NEGATIVE 70

BUT, CHESS,
I DON'T KNOW
WHAT I'M
FEELING! 74

27

I'm feeling fearlessly <u>BRAVE</u>

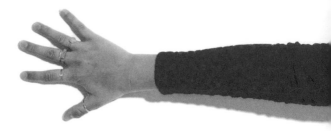

MY DEFINITION: the red lipstick of emotions. You're walking round with a big old 'I was brave at the dentist' sticker on your forehead and you feel like you could tick off every task on every to-do list you've ever made.

This **surge** of energy can come when you least expect it, but **how super-fucking-duper does it feel**? For me, I get this rush of power after a coffee or a matcha! Other times, it's post-workout (or post-orgasm) – all those endorphins rushing through my body like electricity. The docs and specialists out there know that dopamine and oxytocin improve brain function, they flush out cortisol (the stressy bits). For me, I like to think of it as brain food – my mind is feeding off those chemicals, creating ideas, and I feel invincible.

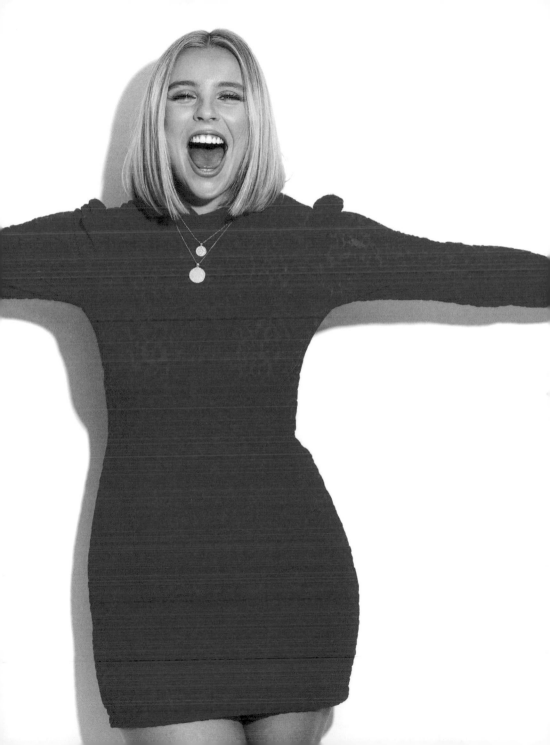

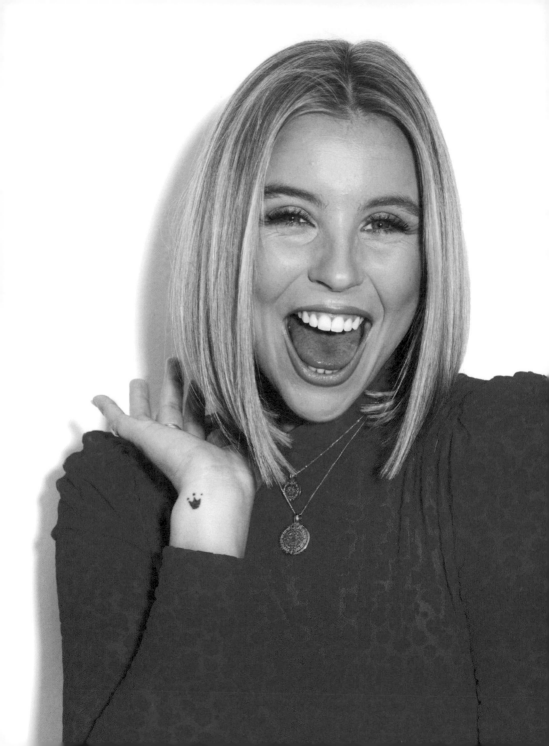

You know those massive inflatable sumo suits, or those huge zorb balls you can climb into? Well, when I was 19, I had to go into the Houses of Parliament actually dressed in one of those. Yes, I was a human 'hive' for Allergy Awareness Day. I had to be rolled through the door lengthways, with my legs poking out the end, as I couldn't fit through standing. When I feel superpowered, I feel like **this** – like I'm wearing **armour**, an inflatable shield of invisibility; I'm protected and I can do anything. We are our own secret weapons when we're feeling courageous.

When I started doodlin' and designing my own prints, I just did it for me, in my notebook. I absolutely loved the creativity flowing out of my brain and it was super-calming. I've never been 'arty' – I mean, I can draw a pretty inspiring stick woman – but since leaving home at 18, I've always filled my bedrooms with quotes and colourful prints. Around Christmas time 2018, I showed my Future Husband Mat (since finishing this book, Mr Carter has proposed and by the time you read this … we may be married) and my family my notebook scribbles and told them I wanted to make them into something. They encouraged me to do more. One morning I woke up, felt this tingly sensation in my body like I just wanted to pour all my love and every ounce of creativity into what are now my CKret prints – my babies. I just went for it. I kept repeating, 'I've got this.' I didn't have anyone telling me what to do or feeding me the motivation to kick it all off; it was just me, my brain and my cash.

I have worked over 30 different jobs since I was 14, but I had never set up my own business with products that I was hand-designing all by myself. There was so much more to it than just drawing stars and writing a quote about magic. I hired an illustrator, who is just brilliant, and from day one, she just understood me – she transforms my ideas and makes them the **real deal**. So, after finalising the original six prints to start with, I set up the business 42 days after my first scribble. For the first month, I wanted to do it all myself, to fully immerse myself in the business. I wanted it to feel personal, to handwrite a thank-you to the people that believed in me and bought a print. I was doing the designing, the printing, the packing, the personal notes, the shipping labels, the post-office run, the customer service … a month turned into two and I was packing over a hundred orders a day. It was incredible and so unexpected; I had to rally round the troops (my brother Henry, my mumma and postman Mat) to help with the sheer volume.

I look back now and realise it was all because I woke up one day feeling brave, ready to work on something new and take a risk – now **that** was a **superpowered** moment.

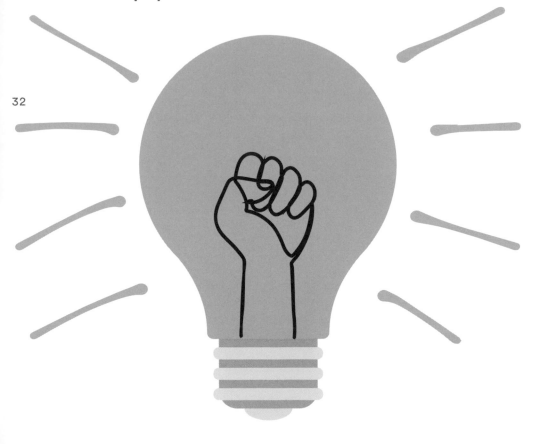

Channel that superpower

So you've got this energy vibrating inside you – let's **do something** with it. This is the perfect time to challenge yourself, to start something new, to say goodbye to self-doubt, to say 'I love you' first, to come out to your parents, to take **risks** …

When I was at school, I couldn't wait for the summer holidays, and to **stop** learning things for eight weeks. But when you're an actual adult, you realise life is so much more exciting when you keep topping up your toolbox of skills, and I'm way more of an interesting human if I'm learning new shit.

A few years ago, instead of making New Year's resolutions, I wrote down five things that I used to do when I was younger that I haven't done since moving to London at 18 (where you're distracted by everything and your monthly rent is the same price as buying a private jet …) and missed.

It was honestly one of the best mini-challenges I set myself and I urge you to do it, too. It doesn't have to be five. These were two of mine.

ROLLERBLADING

The remains of half of my left knee still lives on the concrete pathway in Battersea Park – exhilarating for four minutes until I took a nose-dive into the floor, smashing my phone and nearly my face. Luckily I was with one of the most multi-talented humans to grace this planet. A best friend who doubles up as my regular saviour (while juggling a highly sought-after hand-modelling career), Sammy peeled me off the floor and carried me to the first-aid centre. It was only then, at 22 years old, that I fully understood why Mum always insisted I wore knee pads, wrist pads, a helmet and two pairs of trousers. The scar lives to tell its story, but it honestly made me feel **alive**. It reminded me that the world is our playground.

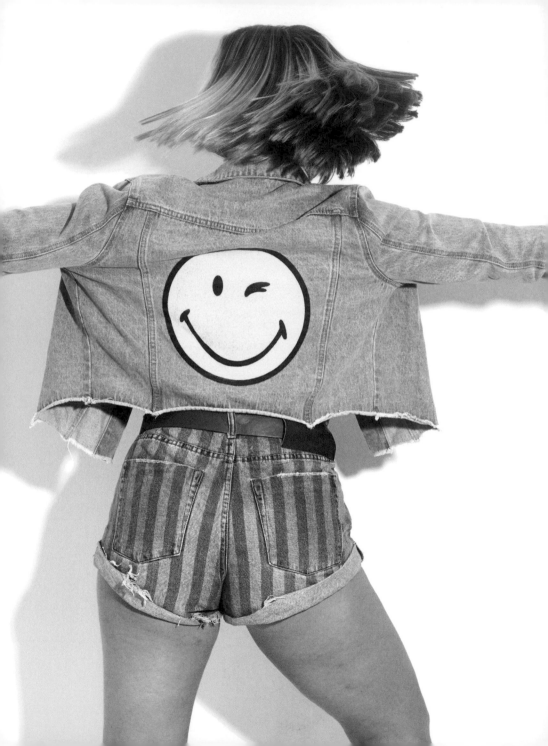

DANCING

I mean, I've never actually stopped. I'm a professional dancing-in-the-house-completely-naked-until-I'm-sweating dancer … but when I was younger, dancing shoes were permanently glued to my feet. My entire out-of-school life was dedicated to it – but in my teens I went from doing eight hours a day, doing shows monthly and regular auditions, to doing nothing in the space of a few weeks. So this challenge gave me the fuel I needed to join my friend Lottie in a dance lesson. Before I knew it, I was lost in the music, prancing away, giving the mirror some fierce looks I didn't even know I had in me … It felt so liberating. During and after, I just felt pure joy.

Finding my inner child re-lit that fire inside of me. I proved that voice in my head wrong and it made me realise that if you stop anything you love, it's not forever. You can always come back to it at a different stage of your life.

What did you do that you haven't done since you were a dinky kiddywink? Swimming? Horse riding? Tennis? Painting? Trampolining? Make a promise to yourself that you'll try at least one of those again in the next month. It might feel new, it might feel like you never stopped. But just know, however it feels, you are never too old. Do it once, do it weekly, but most importantly, do it for **yourself**.

Stretch yourself, believe in yourself, keep filling your brain with new things. It's ironic that as you get older, things become more accessible, but life gets in the way. Give yourself the time your younger self would thank you for. Channel and savour that superpower. Hopefully this offers a little encouragement to give yourself that boost to take this feeling to the next level. I know you are more capable than you think.

I'm feeling <u>PROUD</u>

MY DEFINITION: Your inner cheerleader is chanting, 'Give me an O, give me an H, give me a YAAAAS ... Give me an I. Give me a D. I. D. I. T. And what do you have ... OH YAAAAS, I DID IT!'

Whatever you did, no matter how big or small that thing was, I am so damn proud of you. We're going to celebrate this moment because next time you doubt yourself, you can come back to this place and remember how glorious you felt.

We can all be pretty bad at congratulating ourselves, but giving yourself recognition is so important in building our self-esteem and becoming our own best friend.

I feel so much pride for my friends, family, Mat and total strangers – but I have struggled to congratulate myself in the past. I'm easily proud of the little things like putting on a white wash without turning it all pink by sneaking in a red sock. But with the bigger things, the things other people were 'proud' of me for, I just couldn't feel it. But we're working on it, my best friend and I.

Writing this is genuinely the proudest I have ever felt of myself. Every time I sit down at my laptop to write words, I do a little wiggle. I think it's a real milestone for me, it's a **proud mum** moment, like I'm proud of my brain, proud of my fingers for tap-tap-tapping away.

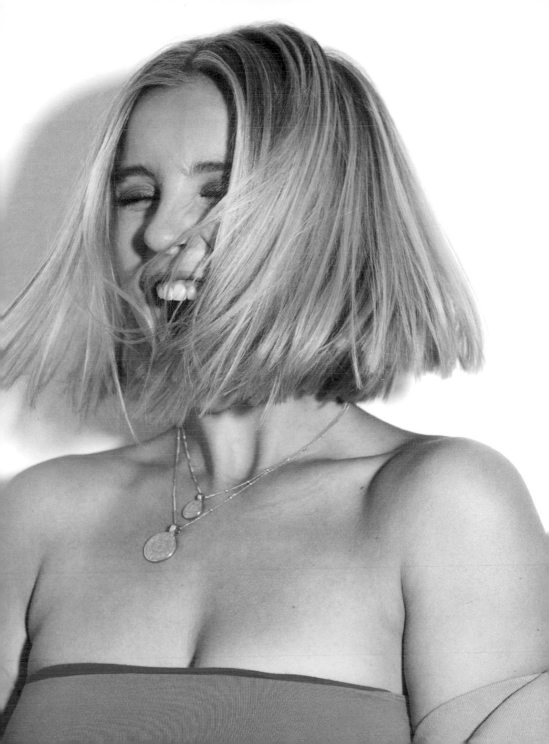

INDULGE IN THIS PRIDE.

Tell your brain just how phenomenal you are. Not anyone else – **you**. This is your time to big up yo-self. It's not just saying, 'Well done, good job gal,' once a year – it's a daily thing, because it all adds up. You have to believe you're worthy of the congratulations, the celebrations. Be your own supporter, cheerer-on-er and then spread the lalalove:

You have three 'I'm proud of you' compliments in your kindness bank; they're to give away today, tomorrow and the next day …

1. For you

WHAT ARE YOU PROUD OF TODAY?

Write it down – you can read this whenever you're stuck in a patch of self-doubt. Revisit it, relive it.

38

HEY ME. REMEMBER THAT TIME YOU …

did your first talk at a school and spoke to 150 girls about body confidence, mental-heath awareness and social media?

YOU ORIGINALLY THOUGHT THAT …

you wouldn't be able to do it, so you were

going to say no when you were asked to speak
for an hour on your own.

so appreciated and you still buzz off the energy
in that room now. You woke up the next morning
so proud of yourself, you were paid in hugs,
lovely feedback and teachers who said how
interesting they found the talk.

SEE, YOU CAN DO IT.

2. For a stranger

I see you – you're feeling yourself, let's use that rocket fuel to make someone else feel proud of themselves too. Let's show everyone else some love and feed them some of your energy. You've noticed the new assistant in the office is feeling a little anxious as it's her first day – give her that extra boost and recognition she deserves by commenting how well she did when you're leaving the office. Build each other up, see people, hear people, root for each other. A fire doesn't lose anything when lighting another fire.

3. For a family member/friend/ partner/colleague

With all compliments, they should come from a place of truth, and not just be forced, because that won't help anyone.

See how it goes down … how do they take it? If they deflect it, say it again in a different way … I find rephrasing it works – mean it and repeat it:

'Bianca, that article you wrote was so interesting.'

'It wasn't my best. I could've done much more research if I had the time.'

'Honestly, I found it fascinating. Believe me and believe in yourself.'

It's never too late for you to start being proud of yourself – it doesn't mean you're 'cocky' or 'arrogant'. Come back to this joyful feeling when your inner cheerleader has gone quiet on you.

BELIEVE YOU'RE A BADASS.

I'm feeling <u>HONEST</u>

MY DEFINITION: when you feel like it's time to be totally truthful with yourself AND with others.

This is your time to come clean; you're ready to open up and say it how it is. I'm writing this bit with my bits out … I'm completely naked. I ran out of the shower to do this little section – it came to me just as I was washing my armpits.

TRUTH-FACED OR TWO-FACED?

As I've grown up, I've learnt that the more open and honest I am with my friends, the stronger and more understanding our relationship is. Especially for women, there is still a stigma around us all being 'two-faced' and not telling each other how we really feel about things … well, that's not how I roll. There is absolutely no benefit to speaking behind someone's back. I believe it's better to address a situation before it becomes a mess – this is what I like to call being 'truth-faced'.

Honesty doesn't have to a brutal – 'Wow, you're totally shit at singing, please stop, I'm sending you the invoice for my broken ear drum surgery' – it can be nurturing and 'character-building'. If anyone has upset me or made me feel uncomfortable, I meet up with them face to face and tell them with kindness and empathy. I know they might not even be aware of it, or they didn't intentionally do it, or they could be going through something.

I have a good friend who I've known for years. We have a very complex friendship, but we respect and understand each other.

Honesty = Trust
Trust = Strength
Strength =
Solidarity

She's admitted that, before me, none of her other friends had ever been honest with her. Out of courtesy, I'm going to call her by another name: Gladys.

Gladys has been through things no human should have to deal with. I cannot even imagine the pain and hurt she's been through and how it has affected her. There was a stage in our friendship where she was spending most of our time together talking about other people negatively. It left me feeling really deflated, questioning whether she spoke about me like that to others ... so I addressed it head-on. I said exactly how I felt, and asked if she was aware she was even doing it. She was initially a little defensive, saying that she didn't mean it maliciously; she was processing stuff and her way of doing that was talking about others, to me.

A few months later, Gladys thanked me for being honest with her. It had made her think and she was more aware of spending time talking about other people while she was with friends. I was genuinely quite surprised by the effect our conversation had had on her, but we are now even closer because of it.

I used to be sensitive to honesty; I was a confrontaphobic. I would immediately go into self-protection mode and make an excuse for myself before apologising. It can be hard to take, but flip it round and be honest with yourself: if you didn't know you had upset a friend, would you prefer them to communicate with you directly or would you want them to go to someone else and talk about you?

I find that if you both have a mutual understanding and level of respect for each other, you will have one conversation about whatever it was and then (hopefully, and I talk about this later in the book) it won't happen again. I believe honesty is a really important part of building a friendship.

Being honest isn't just an emotion you can use with others; it's just as powerful if you use it on yourself.

It can be painful, but these moments leave me feeling empowered – like I'm taking back control of my life and deciding to make a change. It took me a good chunk of time to be honest with myself about a previous relationship that had left me feeling weak and trapped. I felt like someone had smothered me in superglue and stuck me to this relationship for just over a year – I had convinced myself I wasn't strong enough to get out of it. So you don't all go after him, I'm going to call him Hamish – because Mat had a goldfish called Hamish when he was seven, and things with this guy felt **fishy** from the start …

Writing this now and opening locked-up memories actually helps me understand why I'm more apprehensive about self-celebration … every time I came back from work with exciting news, I would always get shot down by his pessimism. This was at a stage of my life when I was shifting jobs, from working at a start-up app in London to getting somewhere with my presenting. I'd come back home late after events, super-excited to share them with Hamish, but he would ask, 'Why would you want to interview these fake people on red carpets?' 'What satisfaction do you get out of this fake industry, with your fake hair, fake nails and fake friends?' Hamish was the king of eye rolls. He was the guy who told me I couldn't do something when everyone around me was trying to show me I could. He was the guy who left me broke at 23, financially (I couldn't afford a £10 dinner out with friends, let alone my rent in London) and mentally. He was the guy who told me I was overreacting when I'd driven back from leaving my nana in hospital after watching her go through a biopsy. He said she was absolutely fine and I was making it sound worse than it was … she died a few days later.

No one really knew what was going on, but people made comments online and in real life about his negativity, especially towards my job. It started becoming more transparent to others how unenthusiastic and disapproving he was of my life. He put me down constantly and had stolen so much of my happiness I didn't feel like myself at all. Friends were noticing it, family could see a slither of it, and I knew I had to get out. Waking up one day and feeling truly honest with myself gave me the extra fuel I needed to end it.

HARNESS IT

So, you're ready to channel your inner honest-truth-faced-Chessie? If you're in a difficult situation with a friend, partner, work colleague or family member, don't let it get worse – let's work through it and hopefully settle things between you.

HERE'S MY STEP-BY-STEP GUIDE ON HOW TO APPROACH IT HONESTLY WITHOUT:

a) hurting them

b) hurting you

c) blowing things up to be bigger than they already are/should be, and

d) protecting the friendship, if, at the end of it all, you want to remain close.

Get a date in.

THE SOONER YOU CAN MEET UP, THE BETTER, SO IT'S NOT BUBBLING AWAY FOR DAYS/WEEKS.
'Morning _____, are you free to meet up this week?
Let's pick up a coffee and go for a walk.'

⬇

WALKS ARE BRILLIANT
for talking about important things – there's something
about walking next to each other that feels free, and you
don't have to stare at each other from across a table. Plus
being outside is always a good idea.

⬇

BUT WHAT DO I SAY?
'I want to be open and honest with you because I really value
our friendship.
The other night/_____ I felt hurt/uncomfortable/
upset_____ when you said _____.
Now, I know you might not have said it maliciously or to hurt
me, but it's been playing on my mind.'

⬇

LET THEM SPEAK.
Listen to their response.

↙   ↘

**ARE THEY
DEFENSIVE?**
Go to page 48

**ARE THEY
APOLOGETIC?**
Go to page 49

1. IF THEY ARE DEFENSIVE
If they don't see where you're coming from,
try one of these two options:

'Look, I really appreciate/love you. I hope you can see where I'm coming from. If I said/did that to you, how would you feel?'

GO TO 2

Ask them to repeat what they said to your face. They might not be able to say it because they might not remember it. Or, if they do, their brain will catch up with them while they are saying it out loud and they will hopefully understand why you felt the way you did (channel your inner Marisa Peer – author, therapist and goddess).

You've said what you needed to say and your friend may not be in the right headspace to take it. If they're a true friend and you've both listened to each other, you may just need time apart to digest it all. People react differently, especially when confronted face to face.

2. IF THEY ARE ACCEPTING/ APOLOGETIC
Your response could be something like:

↓

'Thank you for understanding. I wanted to speak to you about it because I would never want our friendship to be affected if I just held it all in. Thank you for hearing me out. I'm really glad we can be mature about things like this. I believe it makes a stronger friendship.'

I've been through all of the above, but I promise, there's peace in knowing you've listened to yourself. Be proud you trusted your emotions.

PAYOFF:
Honesty can be scary, it can be difficult, but it can also be transformative. It can bring you closer to your friends and to yourself or it can help you distance yourself from people who are making you feel like shit. Always choose talking about it to the person over speaking behind their back.

I'm feeling <u>CALM</u>

MY DEFINITION: Enjoying the magic of being in the moment: the right here, right now, RIGHT HERE, RIGHT NOW … sing it, Fatboy Slim.

In our jam-packed, go-go-go lives, we are constantly thinking: 'What's next?' Our brain goes into overdrive thinking about the future, not the **now**.

I'm guilty of getting worked up thinking of my ridiculously busy day **tomorrow**, which ruins my **today**. Or thinking back to an interview I did a few days ago, replaying it back in my head wishing I hadn't gone in for the second kiss on the cheek afterwards while they were fixed on just the one (something I don't think any of us have mastered – the art of greeting a stranger politely … Is it one? Is it two? Is it five on the cheeks then one on the lips?!).

What I have learnt is that I cannot rewrite the past, but I **can** control how I feel about it.

I still gotta remind myself to slowwwwww the paaaaaceeee dowwwwn. A few years ago, I made myself pretty sick because I just didn't stop. I was on the go constantly, life was **bonkers**. I was saying yes to everything, a yes woman. I was unwell with back-to-back illnesses because my body was just screaming out for me to stop. It was telling me I needed plugging in and recharging after running myself completely empty, but I still wanted more more, more …

Mr Mathew 'Calm' Carter and my zen-filled mother have helped me by installing a very important word in my personal dictionary – **no**.

'Yesterday is history. Tomorrow is a mystery. Today is a gift. That is why it is called the <u>present</u>.'

ALICE MORSE EARLE

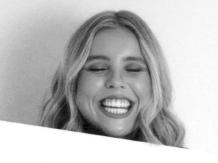

Life isn't as
chaotic and
fast paced
as your brain
makes it out
to be.

With social media comes a lot of performance 'busy'. People are constantly trying to show how much they're working. I'm so used to reading stuff like this on Instagram Stories: 'Wow life has been non-stop madness for 62 weeks, haven't had a second to breathe but my 4am alarm is ready for my morning spin, nine back-to-back meetings, lunch with the CEO of girlbossuniverse.com, **then** I'm hosting an event for 123 of you (last tickets available swipe-up!) while trying to film you a make-up tutorial you've all been asking for, then I'm back to my laptop to #wurkwurkwurk #nodaysoff ...'

Seeing other people being busy does not mean they're more productive than you; it does not mean they're more popular, nor does it mean they're more successful. The most valuable thing we can do is look after ourselves – and that's where we find the power in saying **no**. N. O. Saying stop when everyone else is saying **go**.

Losing my hearing suddenly was a momentous time in my life – which I speak about in Chapter 2, Our Bodies (see pages 144–45) – it has carved out the way I look after myself now and for the future. I feel like a tiny little human found its way inside my brain and installed an internal stop button that I now have full control over. I'm still learning how to find a blend of stillness in the chaotic-ness of my life and how to absorb every moment in the pandemonium. There are still days when I get swept up in my chockablock calendar, but I check in with myself, acknowledge it, and if I need to, do something about it. I think the most powerful tool I've learnt is that we are all in control of this moment, right **now**.

'Mindfulness' is a term that's been chucked around for years, but I never fully appreciated how it feels to be mindful until last year. It sounds like your mind should be full – full of what? Thoughts? But isn't that the opposite of what you're trying to achieve? Well, after trying meditation and finding what works for me, I've realised thoughts are part of 'just being'. Telling your brain to switch off and stop thinking is like telling your lungs to switch off and stop breathing. Have you ever been in a situation or been somewhere with your favourite people, convinced you're having the best time in the world? You're in this bubble like no one else exists and nothing else matters? That's my absolute favourite state of 'just being'. It doesn't always have to be sitting down, with crossed legs, in silence, repeating a mantra in your head.

In the wild world we live in, there's always somewhere to be. There's always someone to see. There's always more to do. It's rare to just BE.

SHARE A PIECE OF YOUR PEACE

Wherever you are in the universe, try something from the list below to put this feeling to use.

When I feel calm and present, I try to use it to help myself and others by:

★ Calling a friend or family member that is going through a difficult time or someone I haven't spoken to in a while.

★ Feeling like I can be completely there for them, giving them my full focus and attention to just **listen** without any distractions.

★ Focusing on a task that has been on my to-do list for weeks. Something I've put off because it seemed too much to even get started on, too mind-boggling, but today I'm ready to tackle it.

★ Simply just taking everything in and soaking up the moment. Those situations where I forget I have a phone, forget I have a meeting next week, forget I'm on my period – just absorbing where I am and what I'm doing. (You're basically doing the job of a tampon, a pad, a menstrual cup/your favourite choice of period protection ... you're just mopping up the moment instead of blood!)

The result? You feel like the bawwwws, the CEO – like you're in control of your life and your life's not controlling you. There are so many places you could be reading this book, but wherever you are, trust that you are right where you need to be.

I'm feeling <u>SWAMPED</u>

MY DEFINITION: when you've got too many tabs open in your brain, you're drowning and life feels like an overwhelming, stressful mess.

Mini Chessie did **all** the activities – at school, after school, on weekends … Life was non-stop, packed with dancing, singing, theatre school, drum lessons, swimming, diving, horse riding, tennis, homework, revising … but it all felt manageable back then because I had Julie taxi-driver King, AKA superwomannnnn. Being an adult is a little bit different! I have those days when I feel like there's a squillion and one things to do, one of me and only 24 hours in the day to get it all done. Sometimes when we're overloaded with the glorious bollocks of life, we have to remind ourselves how much our noggins are doing for us.

Our brains are very good at making things way more serious than they actually are. Don't make your life more exhausting than it already is – it doesn't need to be. If we all stay in this state of 'I have so many things to do and I just can't do it all and if I don't get them done someone's going to die and I feel like it's going to be me', that pressure is going to limit our ability to **get shit done** (short term) and our happiness levels (long term).

Dr Chatterjee (who Mum is only slightly obsessed with … She has his podcasts on repeat and sends every new episode of his to Dad, Brontë, Henry, Mat and I … and her yoga students) talks about 'micro stresses' and how they can all add up to feeling overwhelmed. That feeling when your brain is about to explode might have a little something to do with a morning of micro stresses like this:

★ You snooze your 6 a.m. alarm three times, then check your phone and it's 7.30 …

★ You start reading your 42 million messages, determined to clear your WhatsApp sitting on the toilet.

★ Ten minutes later and you're still sat there even though you finished nine minutes ago because you're trying to reply to your boss's '**Urgent. Please respond ASAP**' email.

★ You turn on the radio, and the news is telling you all your trains are delayed by an hour.

★ You look on Maps to see how long it would take you to walk the six miles to the office … 75 minutes … cute.

★ You click on Instagram just to see how your post went down the night before, then somehow end up on your friend's ex's mum's dog's profile, liking a photo the dog posted in 2014.

★ You get on a replacement bus because your train is now cancelled and realise you left behind your lunch that you spent over an hour packing up last night.

★ You finally get into work at 2 p.m. and your boss calls you in for a meeting to talk about your time management …

I'VE BEEN THERE … I'VE GOOGLED 'CAN A PERSON SELF-COMBUST AND IS IT MESSY?' NO WONDER YOU FEEL CLOGGED UP AND READY TO IMPLODE – YOUR BRAIN IS FULL TO THE BRIM!

LET'S CLOSE SOME TABS DOWN

Our brains were not designed to take on an endless stream of emails, WhatsApps, comments, messages, notifications and constant noise ... You need to give your mind the quiet it needs to sift through all this information.

Tell me what you're thinking about. Grab your notebook and let's have a satisfying brain dump ...

★ Draw your brain – whatever shape, squiggle or outline.

★ Write all the words, all your thoughts, the questions – everything going on inside.

★ Is there anything you **can** answer? Is there anything you can't? Write it down without judgement.

★ What about the things you can control? Ask yourself: is the world going to end if I don't do this? Is anyone going to get hurt? Will it make me happy if I do this?

★ No? No? and No? Well, you don't **have** to do it then. Draw your brain's twin. Empty.

★ Fill it with just three things you **can** do. Three things you **want** to do.

★ Close your eyes and take the deepest breath you can, fill yourself up with air – that air is confidence and belief. Slowly breathe out all the shit you can't control. Know that you can come back to this place, to create space.

Your mind is like a garden,
your thoughts are the seeds,
you can grow flowers,
or you can grow weeds

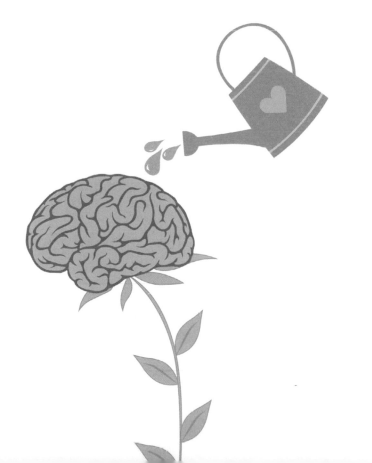

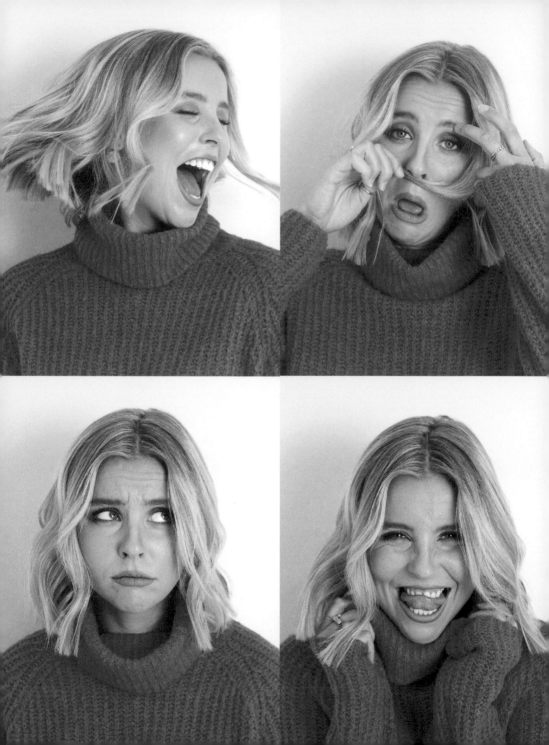

I have always been a yes girl, rarely giving myself time to even think before I've given my answer. But I've learnt how to say **no**. It's a feisty word once you understand its power.

REPEAT AFTER ME:

★ I will say no if someone says, 'Are you okay?' and I'm feeling like shit.
★ I will say no to things that make me feel uncomfortable.
★ I will say no to, 'Are we still on for tonight?' if I don't want to be 'on' for tonight.
★ I will say no to seeing people who make me feel heavy and negative.
★ I will say no to things that aren't going to help me or anyone else.
★ I will say no when I know I need to say yes to looking after myself.

... and never feel guilty for it. Be proud that you made that choice for yourself. You honoured your freeeeeeedom.

The moral of my swampy story: you can do anything ... remember not to confuse that with everything.

I'm feeling <u>NOT GOOD</u> <u>ENOUGH</u>

MY DEFINITION: when your inner critic is loud, you feel heavy with self-doubt and self-destructive thoughts.

I hear you. It's shit but it won't be forever; this is just a feeling and it will pass. I've been through these days/weeks/periods of my life. I felt it this morning while tapping away on my laptop writing this, so I listened, spent an hour looking at puppies, because I really, really want one, and came back when I was ready.

Think of self-appreciation like the Freddo inflation. Who remembers Freddos when the little guys were 10p? Me. Now, I believe they believed they were worth more – they put their prices up year after year. I'm a Freddo – every year my age goes up, my value of myself goes up, too.

I don't think we help ourselves when it comes to hearing compliments from others – I'm convinced most of us are allergic to them. We get all funny when someone shhweet talks us. How many times have you replied to 'I love your dress, the colour is gorgeous on you' with something like 'Really? Oh, well it was super cheap, literally £10 in the sale. It's not even that nice. I think it would look nicer on you – you can have it [strips off], here, take it' … RIP to all the flattery we deflected and neglected .

On top of my own self-doubts and self-deprecation there's a whole lotta criticism that I receive daily online – from strangers, which just heightens the noise in my head telling me I'm not good

you are enough.
you have enough.
you do enough.

you have always
been enough.
you will always
be enough.

enough. I will talk more about Trolly McTrollfaces in Chapter 4, Our Outer Orbit, but I think it's important to share this here, too. They don't deserve the satisfaction of being published in a book, but it needs to be spoken about.

I've been eaten up by the 'haters' and I've felt like the whole world has been against me. I try to use my Instagram to help, support and act as a big-sister figure to those younger than me, and a best friend to those older. I have tried to make it an account that champions individuality while celebrating a sisterhood community. So, when the cyberbullies invade my space, our space, I want to protect my followers from reading these horrible comments, too.

Recently I described it to a friend like this. She had a drawing by her four-year-old niece stuck proudly on her fridge. It was precious to her and made her smile every time she looked at it. I said, 'Imagine if a stranger walked into your house – uninvited – and stole that drawing. They just came into your safe space and robbed some of your happiness, something you treasure, something you're proud of.' That's what it feels like sometimes. Like they've stolen my voice, silenced me.

I appreciate that I open myself up by sharing my life online, and the more Instagram grows, the more judgement I get. But people feel like they know me from watching a few Insta stories or the first three photos on my profile. I've been called things I'd never wish upon anyone and these comments get me the most on days when I'm feeling vulnerable. Scrolling through the hate is a form of self-harm; it's essentially giving the trolls the time and attention that they so desperately crave. I have the control to stop looking, but still I carry on reading these comments from faceless accounts and they worm their way into my brain. These people are clearly so unhappy in their own lives and I genuinely feel sorry for them, but there's absolutely no excuse to be a dick – it's poisonous.

I've trained my brain to quiet the 'you can't do this' voice, the constant doubting, but it still tries to be heard on days when I've been trolled. It can eat away at you and then you start a tsunami of negativity, questioning whether you can do even the smallest of tasks, which can disconnect you from yourself and from others.

STOP DISRESPECTING YOURSELF

If you can't acknowledge your worth, who will? Being your own best friend is believing in yourself and knowing you're a bloody wonderful human with so much to offer the world.

Let's swap THESE   with THESE

'There's someone who could → 'I am that person and I'm do this better than me.'   going to do the best I can.'

65

Sprinkle yourself with a little bit of extra self-belief.
Hold yourself proud and go show 'em, badass.

'Everyone in this room is → 'I deserve to be here and more successful than me.'   I'm not leaving.'

Everyone's probably thinking the same thing. No one is better or worse than anyone, we are all equal and successful in our own ways.

'My to-do list is eternal and   Maybe my to-do list is a I never get to the end of it. → pile of bollocks and I need to I'm useless.'   rip it up and burn it.

Ask yourself: what's been sitting on your to-do list, untouched, for a week? It's clearly not a priority for you right now. (Try the exercise on page 58.)

And please, please remember, you can always reach out, ask for help – don't try to deal with this on your own. Call or message a positive friend, someone who believes in you, and they can help you turn that negative voice right down to zero.

Raise the praise

Next time someone takes the time to give you a compliment, instead of repelling it, take it. Say thank you and embrace it. Nothing else.

Train your brain ...

Damn, you look glowing today!	→	Wow, thank you.
That wasn't easy, but you did it.	→	Thank you so much for recognising that.
You're such a loyal friend.	→	You're so lovely, thank you.
You smashed that workout, so proud of you.	→	That's really kind, thank you.

SCRIBBLE DOWN ALL THE THINGS THAT MAKE YOU SMILE. THE SIMPLER THE BETTER. THEY DON'T NEED TO BE EUPHORIC MOMENTS, JUST LITTLE THINGS YOU TREASURE.

Here are mine

Going home – home to see the family, Bertie my pup and Norman the cat.

Hearing Mat laugh. It's honestly infectious.

Seeing little tiny tots – if there's a baby near me, I'm instantly happy.

Hugo greeting me even if I've just gone for a shower and come back – his wagging tail, his green eyes and little red heart-shaped nose are just so special.

Holding my goddaughter and watching her discover things for the first time.

Going for a walk anywhere that's green.

Being by water – lakes, the sea ... puddles.

The sunset from our kitchen when it's not raining.

The smell of my dad's hair stuff. He's used the same product since I was tiny and it's such a nostalgic smell.

Pizza. Pasta. Popcorn.

Sunday mornings with music blaring through the house.

Knowing you're reading this.

Candles – Mat says we don't need to pay for electricity with the number of candles I have in the house.

Scribbling down quotes/print ideas in my notebook.

Framing my prints and hanging them in our nest.

Mat, Dad and Henry's ability to commentate on any rugby or football game.

Dancing to my feel-guuud playlist (page 77).

Looking at photos and videos of Nana and Papa

Talking about Nana and Papa to keep them alive

Listening to a podcast while I'm getting ready.

Rejoice in your choice...

to celebrate yourself. You thought taking off your bra, unzipping your tight jeans and kicking off your heels after a night out felt good. Well, this, this right here, is your newfound confidence and I think it pretty much trumps any of the above. Here's to a tidal wave of joy.

I'm feeling ... negative
+ <u>OUT OF WHACK</u>

MY DEFINITION: It's HORMONE TIME (MC Hammer's new track, dropping this year) – when our female chemical messengers have invaded our brain space.

So **at least** once a month (normally around my period or just before I ovulate) I host **the** wildest, most ridiculous dinner party ... in my brain. I've basically invited all my rowdy but wonderful friends round – they're all pretty drunk and I'm trying to juggle their needs while entertaining them, without it breaking out into one big **emotional extravaganza**.

I'VE GOT:
Sobbing Sabrina, who's a serious crier when she's had just a sip of red ... she's drunk half a bottle.
Aggy Aggie, who's kicked off at Sabrina for getting mascara tears on her white top when they hugged.
Lethargic Lea, who's tired, over it and the first one to leave.
Frisky Fannie, whose oestrogen is bubbling away, creating wild inappropriate-for-the-dinner-table-sex-fantasy daydreams.
Moody Monika, who's been in a giant strop since she got here and hasn't said a word to anyone all night.

Hungry Hazel, who's eaten all of Sabrina's food (she was too busy crying to notice).

Nervous Nina, who's worried she's upset Monika, whom she's sitting next to, who hasn't spoken to Nina. No one's having a good time, especially **me**.

Since coming off the pill a few years ago, these **hormone hoedowns** have been even **wilder**. Sometimes, I genuinely feel like I've lost control over my emotions – I can go from feeling deliriously on top of the world to crying over a fluffy dog on the Tube. As women, we have to deal with regular hormonal onslaughts, all while trying to remain calm, capable and competent.

A few months ago, I went to a baby show with my best friend Tess. I'd woken up feeling fine, but as soon as I got on the Tube with her, I felt sick, was sweating my sore tits off and feeling out of **whack**.

Every time I saw a bump or a baby in a pram, I wanted to cry. I ate every free taster in the room. I didn't like the way I was speaking to people, but it wasn't me that was speaking, it was the hormones. We were on the way home, and I felt like my whole day had been disrupted by my emotions. I got myself more and more worked up in my head.

Tess knows me so well, so after not hearing from me for 10 seconds (which is a rarity) she asked me if I was okay. I burst into tears, cuddling her bump, in front of the whole carriage. I kept repeating, 'It's so silly, I can't even say it out loud!' She let me cry and have the time to sort through the jumble in my brain. I finally found the words: 'I want to be a mum more than anything and today was more difficult than I thought it would be.' The day after, I came on my period. My cycles go from 36 days to 65 days – I convince myself I'm pregnant every time I'm late for my period. I genuinely think I experience all of the symptoms because I've made it out to be a reality in my brain. I'm basically having a phantom pregnancy every month and then cry when the test is negative. I'll talk more about this in the next section, but I think we all forget what's actually going on inside us when we're **on**. I've done my own reading and research into my cycle and it is honestly so empowering to learn about it. I've been hooked on the facts and the way we can work with it, not against it.

HELP IT

Let's get that notebook out again: your sidekick. Think of your emotions as your friends; let's untangle and personify them. Just like my full-blown hormone dinner party, imagine them all sitting around a table in your mind.

Draw that table, whatever shape you think it is.
How many emotions have you felt today? Count them out.
Draw that number of little circles around the table.
Write your emotions in the circles – they're your friends.

NAME THEM...

Go through the emotions and what helps you when you're feeling each of them.
Write these all inside the table.
Pull up a chair, sit down and take whatever you wish from the table, whenever you need to.

SERVE YOURSELF FIRST, THEN SERVE YOUR FRIENDS.

On days when you feel like your hormones are in charge, give yourself a little bit of extra time to react to things, to people and to yourself.

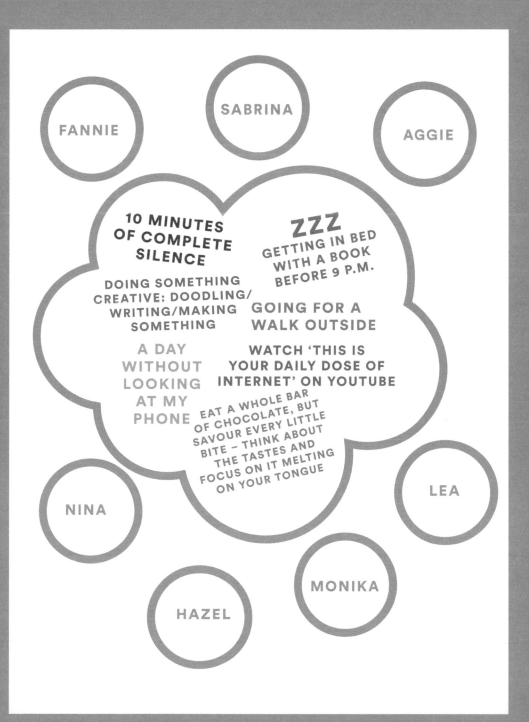

FANNIE

SABRINA

AGGIE

10 MINUTES OF COMPLETE SILENCE

ZZZ GETTING IN BED WITH A BOOK BEFORE 9 P.M.

DOING SOMETHING CREATIVE: DOODLING/ WRITING/MAKING SOMETHING

GOING FOR A WALK OUTSIDE

A DAY WITHOUT LOOKING AT MY PHONE

WATCH 'THIS IS YOUR DAILY DOSE OF INTERNET' ON YOUTUBE

EAT A WHOLE BAR OF CHOCOLATE, BUT SAVOUR EVERY LITTLE BITE – THINK ABOUT THE TASTES AND FOCUS ON IT MELTING ON YOUR TONGUE

LEA

NINA

MONIKA

HAZEL

I'm feeling ... <u>BUT,</u> CHESS, I DON'T KNOW WHAT I'M FEELING!

You know yourself better than anyone. So you know when you're not feeling yourself.

I stood under a shower at 11.30 one night recently, uncontrollably sobbing, producing more water from my eyeballs than the actual shower head itself ... the week had got me real good. Everything had just weighed me down and my brain was desperate to release and empty it all. I wrapped myself up in my towel like I would do to a little child coming out of a bath.

I wiped away my tears and told myself I was okay, like nothing had happened. I was going to jump into bed with Mat like everything was absolutely fine. But then I caught myself and asked myself why. Mat is so supportive, so empathic and so understanding – why was I going to lie to him?

I'm aware that I have this strange reaction – it's like any time I cry or feel sad without any solid reason, I feel a sense of guilt. Even typing this out makes me feel like I need to justify my cry, because I'm thinking, 'I know there are so many people in the world going through so much worse than me ... I'm fortunate to live the life I do.' But none of us should compare our feelings to others. It's not a competition between who feels the worst, who's the biggest crier. All of our feelings are valid: they're relative to us and what we're going through.

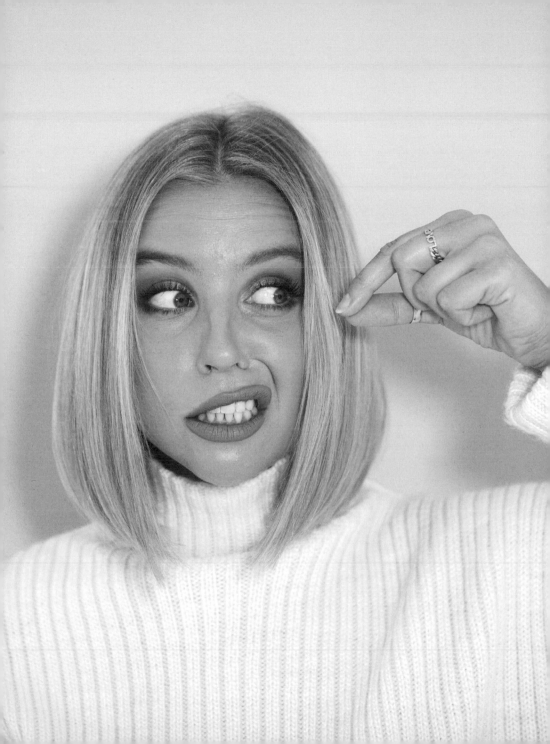

I looked in the mirror at my bloodshot puffy eyes, and told myself I was going to be honest. I walked in and Mat immediately asked, 'What's wrong?' Well, you know when someone asks you if you're okay or what's wrong – then you cry even more, right? (Big girls **do** cry … thanks, Fergie.)

My words were hardly audible, and I erupted, 'I don't even know … I've felt on the verge of exploding all week but I haven't said anything to anyone and now it's all pouring out.' We talked through everything, and things I thought I'd resolved in my brain over the week were still left bubbling away. Mat allowed me to feel sad, he allowed me to talk about it all without any judgement; he helped me untangle the mess I had created in my head all week. It helped Mat open up, too – he'd been feeling 'off' all week, but didn't want to make too much of it because he knew I had so much on. We both went to sleep feeling calmer, reassured, like we'd both shared secrets with each other.

You don't have to know what you're feeling, nor am I saying we have to give all our feelings a specific 'name' or label. All I want you to know is, it feels so much better when you talk about it all when you first feel it, not a week later … even if you don't fully understand what on earth is going on inside you. This is temporary, not forever.

Letting all that emotion build up is like a really tense game of Jenga – it all comes down to that final block being pulled out and everything coming crashing down. If you're that tall, wobbly tower of wooden blocks, put your hand on this page, take three of the deepest breaths you have ever taken (I've just taken them with you with my hand on my laptop screen, so I hope you can feel me with you), and let's stop lying to ourselves, telling ourselves we're absolutely fine.

LET'S PUMP YOU UP WITH GOODNESS

… and get you back in the groove of thangs, by moving our bodies and waking up those endorphins (and you're absolutely not stepping foot in a gym). Put on your favourite song or, if you need a little inspiration, choose one from my **feel-guuud playlist** below. (If you are hard of hearing or deaf, please google these lyrics; they are really powerful and have the same effect from reading them.)

Turn it up (wear headphones if you have stroppy neighbours), dance in your bedroom, living room, kitchen, wherever … Close your eyes, let loose, take your clothes off, keep them on, feel the music, feel the freedom, listen to the lyrics, sing along, make sounds, do whatever the wiggle you need to do.

MY FEEL-GUUUD PLAYLIST

'I Feel Good' – James Brown
'Let Me' – Sérgio Mendes
'Don't Stop Me Now' – Queen
'Walking on Sunshine' – Katrina and the Waves
'Souvenirs' (feat. Zara Kershaw) – Etherwood
'Good as Hell' – Lizzo
'I'm Still Standing' – Elton John
'Ego' – Beyoncé

Our Wo-manifesto

We've reached the end of our Emotional Exploration, so together let's celebrate our glorious, unique worlds with a promise to ourselves.

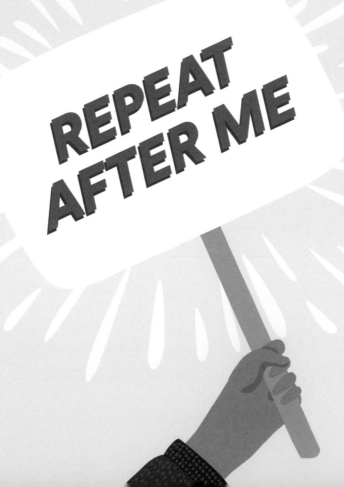

REPEAT AFTER ME

I promise I will celebrate my wonderful, complex self.

I am a three-dimensional, million-dimensional female.

My feelings are valid, I will listen to them, harnessing or helping them when I need to.

I have control over my thoughts and how I react to them, even when it feels like I don't.

I will ask for help when I need it; I will be supported by my solar support system or by a professional.

I will celebrate my unique qualities daily (write yours down in your notebook).

HERE ARE MINE:

I have so much love to give — to my family, Mat, my best friends, the world and myself.

I'm a very good listener.

I try to add sunshine to people's days.

I'm honest with myself and with others — and I'm open to honesty.

My arms are always open for a cuddle/hug/ massive squeeze.

ONE FINAL LITTLE BIT OF LOVE BEFORE WE ZOOM OUT ...

No one at my funeral is gonna say, 'Oh we loved Chessie, she had the perfect nipple-to-boob ratio and her legs were longer than my to-do list.' People are not going to remember us for how we look; they're here for all the yummy stuff inside us. I hope this chapter has left you feeling empowered and you've had the time to celebrate and understand what's going on beneath the surface.

Have you ever received a message from an engineer or a parcel delivery saying you have to be in the house from 4 a.m. to 6 p.m. to sign for it? (Sure, **give me a 14-hour window, I've got absolutely nothing else to do with my life**). Well, I kinda think that's like our feelings, emotions and definitely our hormones. You're expecting them, but who knows when they'll come knocking? You've filled your toolbox up with all the gear to harness and help you, and when they do arrive, I want you to come back to this section and use it however you need to.

RIGHT, ARE WE READY TO ZOOM OUT FROM OUR INSIDES TO OUR OUTSIDES ... OUR BODS?

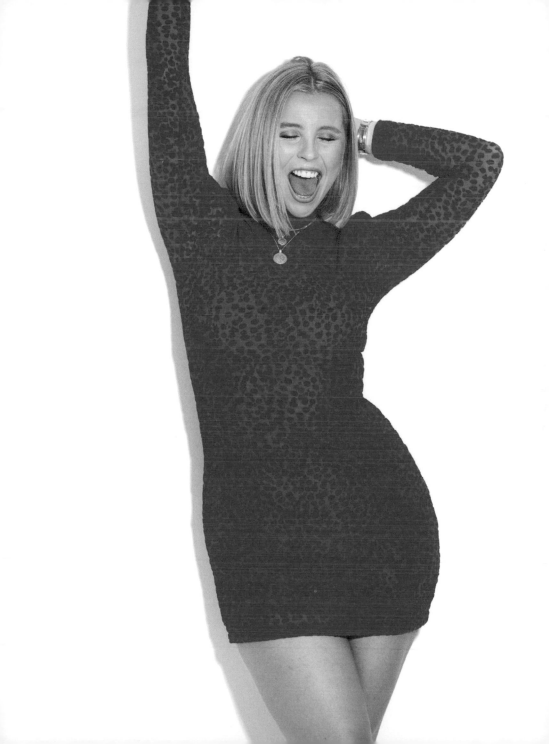

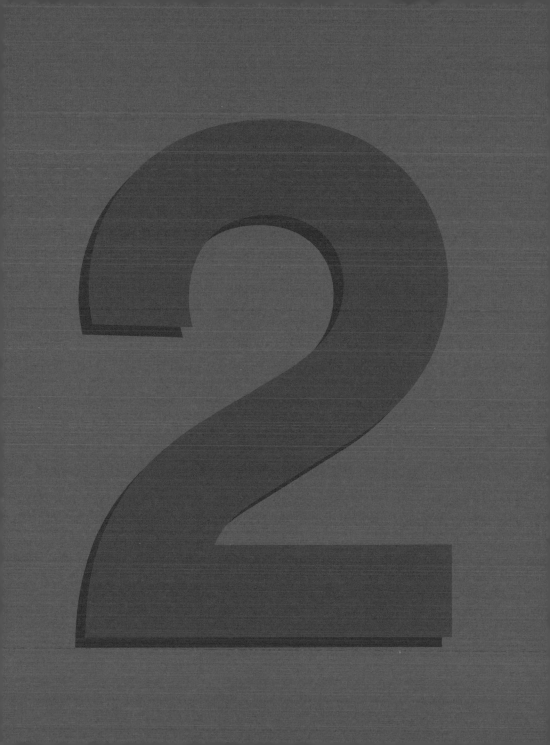

OUR BODIES

SEX, JUGS AND BODY ROLLS

OUR BODIES

This is dedicated to your body, my body, everybody's body: how they change, how they feel, what they do for us and how we can develop a unique, eternal friendship with them …

When I was a little human, I never thought of my body as anything but a useful attachment to my head that allowed me to do whatever I wanted. My body was a dancer at parties playing musical statues; my body was a runner chasing friends around the playground; my body was a swimmer after school in the pool … I was ferociously confident in my body, as every child **should** be. All I wanted to do was explore, make people smile and run around nudey-rudey (a day fully clothed from morning to evening was a rarity … and even then, there are endless photos of me flashing my nappy). Throughout my whole childhood I was lucky enough to feel free and happy in my able body.

But our bodies go through so many changes during puberty, many of which we weren't warned about. No one told me I was going to sweat dark circles that protruded from my armpits in my grey school shirt; no one told me my nipples would start sprouting dark hairs; and even when my mumma told me I was going to start my period, I wasn't quite expecting the amount of monthly maintenance that comes with it.

Over the years, I've been through a labyrinthine journey of body-image bollocks. I was always the tallest out of the girls in my year, I had a mass of body hair and I never felt like I measured up to the ideal image. But in all of that, I've found a deep appreciation and kinship for my body.

I never thought I'd escape the trap of wanting to 'look good naked' – a phrase chucked around the diet culture world. But I can honestly say, I am so full of admiration for my body and all the incredible things it does for me. My fingers are typing this all so fast because I genuinely want to stand on the top of every single building and scream: '**Your bodies are phenomenal, every single last one of them**!' I hope through sharing my little stories and giving you the space to think, I help you realise how fan-bloody-tastic you are. I'm here in these pages rooting for you, believing in you and giving you permission to see you and your body's **worth**.

MY PRIORITIES IN LIFE BEFORE PUBERTY

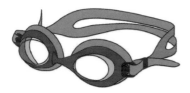

Keeping my rabbit's hutch clean.

Cat's cradle.

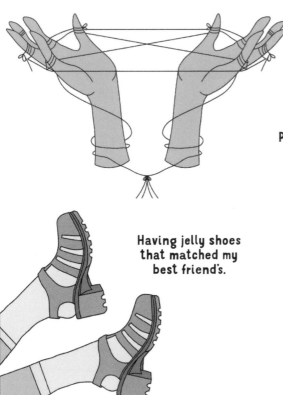

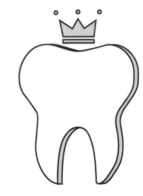

Putting my teeth under my pillow and waking up with £1 – go on, tooth fairy!

Having jelly shoes that matched my best friend's.

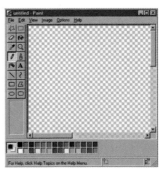

Doing my homework on Paint.

Finding
sweets at
Nana and
Papa's house
before Brontë
and Henry did.

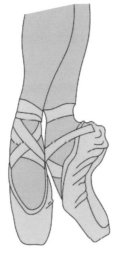

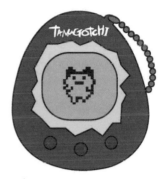

Keeping my
Tamagotchi
alive and
my Furby quiet.

Collecting
Beanie
Babies.

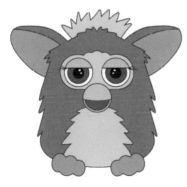

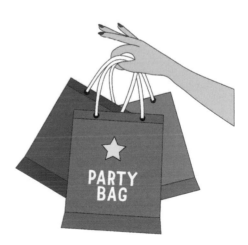

PARTY
BAG

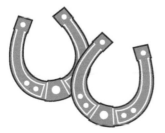

Party bags

MY PRIORITIES IN LIFE DURING PUBERTY

Trying to work out what all these 'bases' are and what they mean ...

Txtin in the shrtst frm pos & lrnin evry acronym. G2G. BRB.

Finding a way to get rid of all this hair sprouting everywhere.

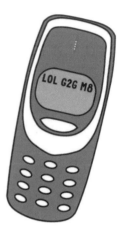

LOL G2G M8

Wondering why on earth I ruin every single pair of pants when I'm on my period.

Making rock-solid plans for my future self. Of course, I'll be married at 23. Baby at 25 ... ninth baby at 32 ...

CHESSIE'S FUTURE PLANS

1. Married at 23
2. Baby at 25
3. Ninth baby at 32

Getting to Blockbuster before it closes to rent a video.

Getting back from school, logging straight on to MSN, Bebo and Myspace before my parents call someone on the house phone and interrupt my dial-up internet connection.

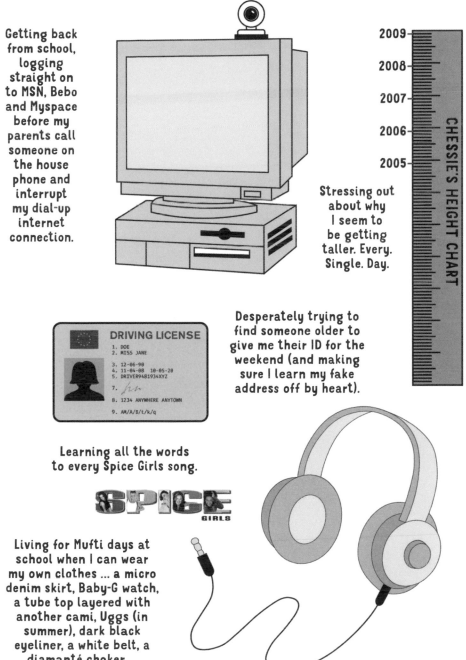

Stressing out about why I seem to be getting taller. Every. Single. Day.

2009
2008
2007
2006
2005

CHESSIE'S HEIGHT CHART

DRIVING LICENSE
1. DOE
2. MISS JANE
3. 12-06-90
4. 11-04-08 10-05-20
5. DRIVER94B1934XYZ
7.
8. 1234 ANYWHERE ANYTOWN
9. AM/A/B/t/k/q

Desperately trying to find someone older to give me their ID for the weekend (and making sure I learn my fake address off by heart).

Learning all the words to every Spice Girls song.

SPICE GIRLS

Living for Mufti days at school when I can wear my own clothes ... a micro denim skirt, Baby-G watch, a tube top layered with another cami, Uggs (in summer), dark black eyeliner, a white belt, a diamanté choker ...

MY PRIORITIES IN LIFE AFTER PUBERTY

Dealing with an endless stream of notifications — emails, WhatsApps, messages, comments.

Realising that timeline I set my future self was hilarious as I sail past all the 'deadlines'.

Obsessing over food — overeating, undereating and sometimes never eating.

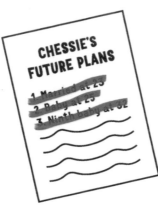

CHESSIE'S FUTURE PLANS
1. ~~Married at 25~~
2. ~~Baby at 25~~
3. ~~Ninth baby at 32~~

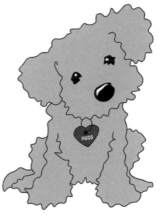

Exploring the difference between sex, making love and everything in between.

Discovering my true, forever-and-ever friendships.

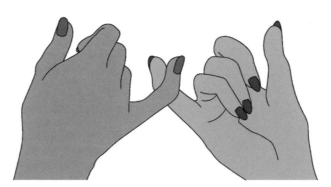

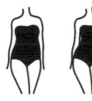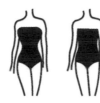

Changing my body for the world, for boys, for myself, for work.

Making money for myself, while simultaneously spending it all on London rent ...

Finding my voice on social media: transitioning from Myspace to Facebook to Instagram ...

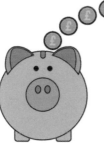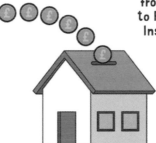

Moving out of home at 18 and lapping up the freedom (while trying to fend for myself).

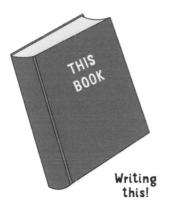

THIS BOOK

LONDON

Writing this!

Finally working out how to get from A to B in London without getting lost.

...oh and trying to live, be a nice human and look after myself

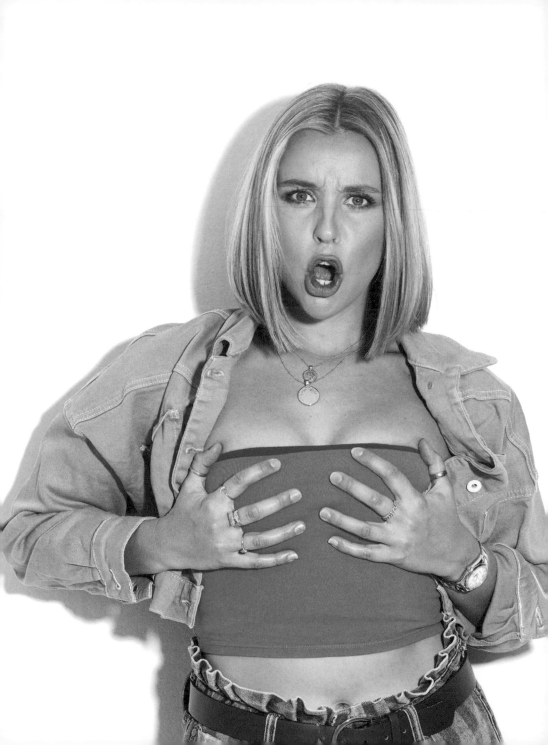

OH. MY. BOD.

Me and my boobies

Boobs. Chestickles. The girls. Melons. Baps. Puppies. Udders. Jugs. Tig ol' bitties. Bazookas. Lovely jubblies. Knockers. Rack. Air bags. Boob-baes.

I was 11 and everyone around me wanted them. They were in higher demand than the new Motorola flip phone. They were cooler than completing level 96 on Snake. They were better than the latest Baby-G watch … and those of us who weren't graced with them early on tried *all* the tricks. When I couldn't steal my mum's padded bra, I wore two of my unpadded ones. I'd heard if you squeeze your hands together in a clasped prayer over and over again, they'd start blowing out. A friend told me her sister was on the 'boob diet'. Uh-huh. Who knows what she was eating on that.

When they came, they were **fascinating**. I couldn't believe my body was growing them. It was like walking around school with a gold medal around my neck, but being told to wear the medal underneath my jumper, where no one was allowed to see it.

Thirteen-year-old Chessie was thrilled with her new friends, making sure every photo contained a lot of boobage – as my dad would say, I was 'oversharing'! I was tits-deep in love but completely oblivious to their biological role – that hopefully one day they will feed my teeny tiny baby oranges. The novelty of having them wore off after a year or two and they just became part of me, a part of me that I've always loved. They have a tendency to change size quite often, probably due to the number of different contraceptive pills I've been on, and my 'righty' has always been a squish bigger.

I grew up talking a lot about breasts – my nana had a mastectomy after fighting breast cancer at 44. My mumma watched her go through it all when she was 18, so she was aware of the importance of self-examining and passed that on to me and my sister. I've had two 'scares' where I've found lumps, gone to get them checked out pretty quickly, to be reassured they've just been swollen glands or a build-up of tissue. Breast cancer awareness charity Coppafeel are incredible and continue to feed us all with invaluable information.

I try to use my platform to encourage everyone – women, men and non-binary followers – to check their boobies. So, I'm going to use this book to do the same thing. In honour of those we've lost, the warriors still fighting, the survivors … When you're in the shower tonight or tomorrow morning, I want you to feel, inspect and pay attention to your breasts. If you find anything that you don't think feels right, go see your GP and see a specialist.

I appreciate my healthy, squishy boobies every day. They keep my hands warm when I'm cold. They make me laugh when I lie down and they splay out to the sides. They're decorated with mini lightning-bolt stripes from growing with me.

As much as I love them, as I've become older the more I try to cover them up when I'm in public. A few years ago, I'd been presenting at a red-carpet event, it was 11 p.m. and Uber was at a silly surge price, so to get home would've cost me more than the £50 fee for my night's work. I jumped on the Tube, aware I was fairly dressed up for a Thursday night and regretting not packing a more 'travel-friendly' outfit to change into. My dress was floor-scraping (always rare to find for my 6-foot-tall bod) with a scoop neck. I wrapped a scarf around my shoulders for warmth and stood holding onto the pole. A twentyish guy stepped into the carriage at the next stop, looked at the row of free seats, but then looked over to me.

CHECK 'EM OUT

LOOK
Changes in skin texture

LOOK
Swelling in armpit or collarbone

FEEL
Lumps and thickening

FEEL
Constant, unusual pain

LOOK
Nipple discharge

LOOK
Sudden change in size or shape

LOOK
Nipple inversion and direction change

LOOK
Rash or crusting of nipple or areola

for more information and advice visit www.coppafecl.org

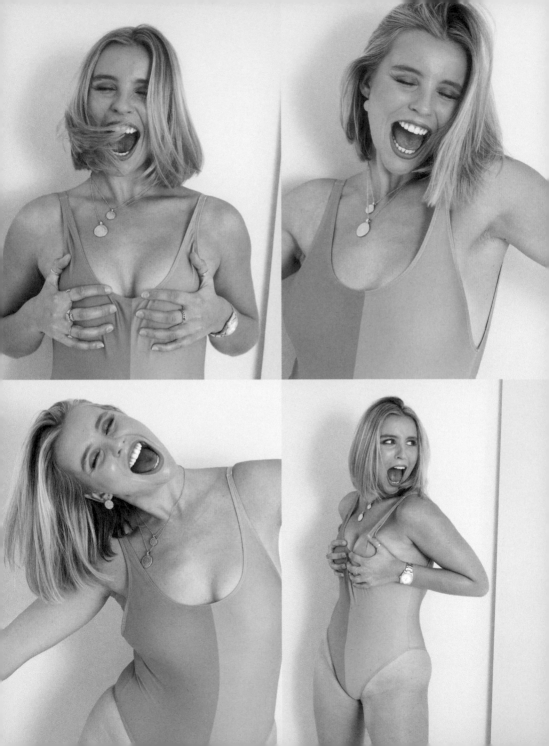

He stood so close I could smell his eau de alcohol married with the stench of stagnant smoke. I felt uncomfortable, so sat down on a chair next to an older woman on her own. The man sniggered, aware I'd moved because of him. Eyeroll. He grabbed the pole by my side, towering over, dominating the space, looking down on me. When I didn't give him any attention, he started shuffling his feet, making sounds and fumbling in the pockets of his baggy trackies. I honestly thought he was about to pull out a weapon. It was his phone, and as soon as the flash went off, I knew exactly what had happened. He staggered off at the next stop, with a photo of me, from above, looking down my dress. I felt superglued to my seat, trapped, alone, like he had just stolen a part of me and taken it with him.

I felt sick from that moment until I woke up the next morning, replaying the situation, going through the different ways I could've taken control. I kept wishing I'd taken a jumper with me and worn it home. All I could think about was his dirty fingers zooming in on my boobs, sending it to his friends (if he had any). My 19-year-old self thought she was feisty back then, but now I realise no matter how 'strong' you think you are, you don't know how you're going to react in those situations – and whatever you're wearing does **not** give people the right to make you feel frightened for your safety.

There will be people who think your body is public property, but **no**. It is **yours**. Every single part of **your** body is **yours**.

No one else's.

So let's start with getting to know our boobs.

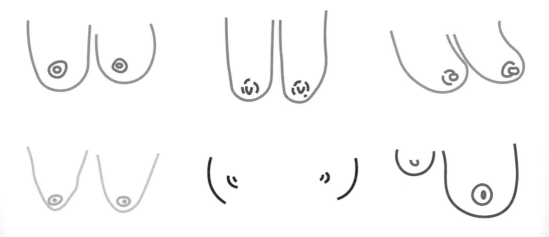

BE BEST FRIENDS WITH YOUR BOOBIES

My boobies are two of my best friends, even though they look like they've had an argument between them (they seem to get further and further apart from each other but closer and closer to tucking under my armpits). The girls have little zigzags on them, their eyes (my nipples) get a little crusty at times and they are the proud owners of little hairs sprouting outta them. They've had a catalogue of names – Meghan and Harry are a new addition to the list. The right one is Harry because, just like Mat's nipples, there were a few ginger strays growing the other day. They get suuuuuuper sore, tender and a little bit lumpy in the week leading up to my period and then throughout, so I give them an extra bit of love and support when they need it.

What stories do your boobies hold? Do you ever look down at them and wish they could talk? (I reckon they speak to each other.) Are they painted with a unique and beautiful tapestry of scars?

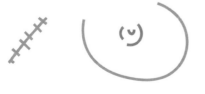

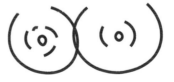

THE MAGIC OF OUR BREASTICKLES

If only we knew ...

★ There is absolutely zilch you can do to make your breasts grow bigger or smaller.
★ It's completely and utterly normal to have inverted nipples, hair surrounding them, stretch marks and lopsided boobies.
★ Our breasts are made up of fatty tissue and ligaments – there are no muscles in them but there are muscles lying underneath them.
★ The parts of our breasts that produce milk are called lobules (cute).
★ Your nipples can get darker during pregnancy. This is Mother Nature's way of making sure your hungry bubba can see the bullseye, as they're colour-blind.

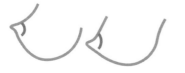

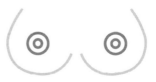

Me and my body hair

Oh hairy-mother-of-Hagrid, we have had a turbulent relationship. I put the pube in puberty. There was just so much of it and I used to think body hair was my **nemesis**. It invaded my skin, starting on places my mum had told me it would be, which even then I wasn't quite ready for, but then sprouting in places I wasn't even aware I had.

Since then, I have pretty much shaved/plucked/whipped off/ removed every single strand from the neck down (I also went through a stage of cutting my own hair, which always ended in tears!). No matter how many times I got rid of the hairy fighters, they always came back even darker, even longer, seemingly even thicker. At school, all my friends were doing it, so I thought it was the only option.

As I was the oldest, Mum was my 'big sister', and although I knew I could speak to her about things, I really should've **listened** to Scrumma King, because she knew her shit. When I was 12, she told me not to shave above my knee because once I got rid of the light, fluffy hair, it would come back darker on the top half of my leg.

So what did I do? I shaved above my knee and it did exactly what she said it would.

She also advised me to just trim my bikini line rather than taking the whole lot off. Instead of listening to her sensible words of wisdom, I took my inspiration from seeing my first ever nudey-rudey hairless vagina in one of my friend's older brother's porn mags. Initially my friends and I laughed at the picture – why did she want to look like we all did BP (before puberty)? Surely pubic hair meant you were a big girl, all grown up? No, apparently being an adult meant you were a pube-less goddess, with fewer things to get 'in the way' of your flower.

I remember once coming home crying after the boys had told me my arms were hairier than theirs and I looked like Sully from

Monsters, Inc. That night, I shaved my **entire** body (except my head, eyebrows and nostril hair … although I tried plucking that out and cried at the first strand, so stopped). I dedicated a whole evening to it. Armed with a blunt razor, I started on my tash, moved down to my chest, up to my armpits, belly button to vagina, in between my peach cheeks, the tops of my legs all the way down to my toes … **Please, please, please do not try this at home**. I was going to see a boy I liked, and thought I needed to be a member of the hair-free society. I'm sure he was convinced I had crabs, as I not-so-subtly itched my prickly pear the. whole. night.

Why, Chess? Why?! How did I convince myself my own body hair was my nemesis? Even though I knew the choice was there to leave it and let it grow naturally, as a teenager I was definitely affected by the boys in my year. They'd already named my 'snail trail' (the hair connecting my belly button down to my lady garden), and they influenced a lot of my choices. But there was also a constant comparison to other girls' bald arms and legs … I brainwashed myself into believing that I wasn't 'normal', I was **too hairy**.

Isn't it funny that when you're younger, you want to grow hair down there to prove you're a teenager and not a girl any more? Then as soon as you hear 'eww, pubes are gross' you want to whip it all off! We're told body hair is unattractive and it should be eradicated. It wasn't until I was at least 22 that I realised I had a choice; I had the freedom to do whatever I wanted with my hair.

Just like everything you do with your body, it's your choice. It feels super-liberating to take back control and do it for myself, not for the boys that I was trying to impress. I'm a firm believer that I was not put on this earth to please the penis. I'm done with pruning my lady garden, I've had enough of the red lady bumps and the itch that comes with it, laser it is …

Be BEST FRIENDS with your hair

CHESSIE'S BODY HAIR MAP

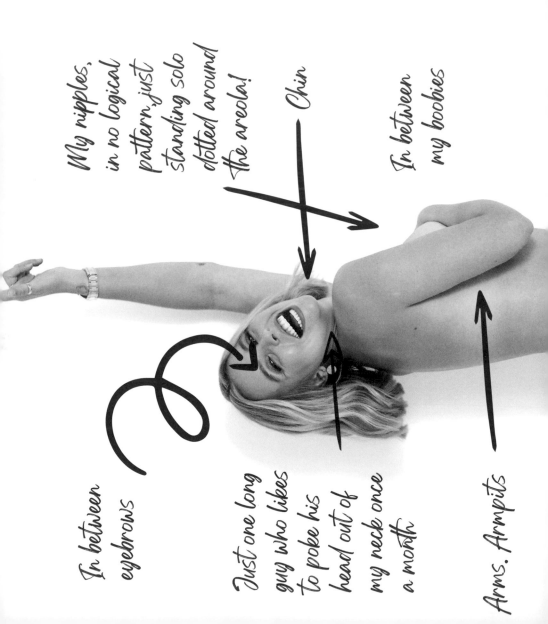

My nipples, in no logical pattern, just standing solo dotted around the areola!

Chin

In between my boobies

In between eyebrows

Just one long guy who likes to poke his head out of my neck once a month

Arms. Armpits

THE TRUTH ABOUT BODY HAIR

We've been fed so many images and ideas that body hair is somehow gross – it's not. It's functional and is there for a reason: it preserves the skin underneath and acts as a barrier to bacteria. It also facilitates sweating, which cools your body. **Go on, hair, you do your thang**.

Belly button to vag

Pubes

Legs

Big toe (but not on any of the other toes)

Me and my skin

My skin and I went to war years ago – and
we've only made up pretty recently.

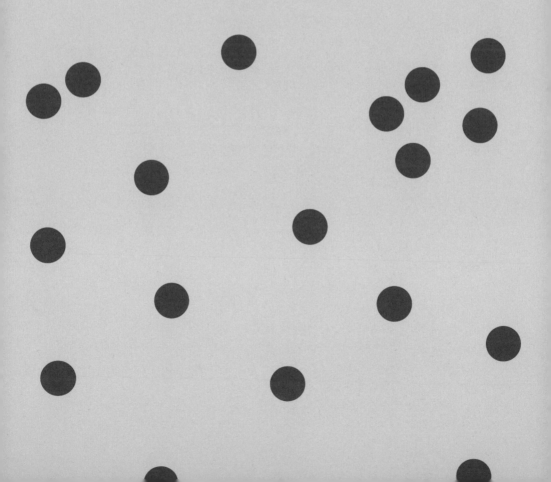

I managed to dodge acne up until I was 17, so when it came I was shocked. It honestly felt like I went to sleep one night, then woke up with the world's most complicated dot-to-dot. I struggled for eight years – I tried **everything**, from eating three raw garlic cloves every morning for a week (until everyone started walking 2 metres ahead and couldn't hold a conversation with me for longer than 10 seconds) to a strong course of Roaccutane, which ate up all the happy cells in my brain (going on medication for six months was my final option, after I'd ticked off every other alternative). My spots were squatters – living on my face without paying rent but refusing to leave.

Deeply embarrassed, I felt like everyone was looking at me as if I was dirty, which was ironic because I was cleaning my face more than three times a day. My cheeks were swarms of red, painful, itchy lumps. The sore clusters even made it hard to sleep lying on a pillow. I did everything to try to hide them: using every concealer ever invented, talking to people with my hair covering my face, making sure I organised meetings or dates in dark places with no natural light. They were so bad when I was 18, I didn't leave the house for three days – I shut myself off from the world, only allowing my family to see me with layers of foundation on. One of my best friends surprised me with a visit, and as I went to give her a hug, she backed off and said, 'Wow, I didn't realise it was *that* bad.' (That *did not* help.)

When I thought it was finally clearing up and we'd called a truce my spots came back for a reunion tour. The course of strong drugs had left me totally **dry** – they had literally sucked up every drop of moisture from my skin. My face was peeling, my lips were permanently crusty, I was shedding layers and layers of skin everywhere. A specialist told me to log it all in a 'skin diary', and I look back on those photos when I'm having a breakout now. My mum, like always, supported me, trying to help me find a

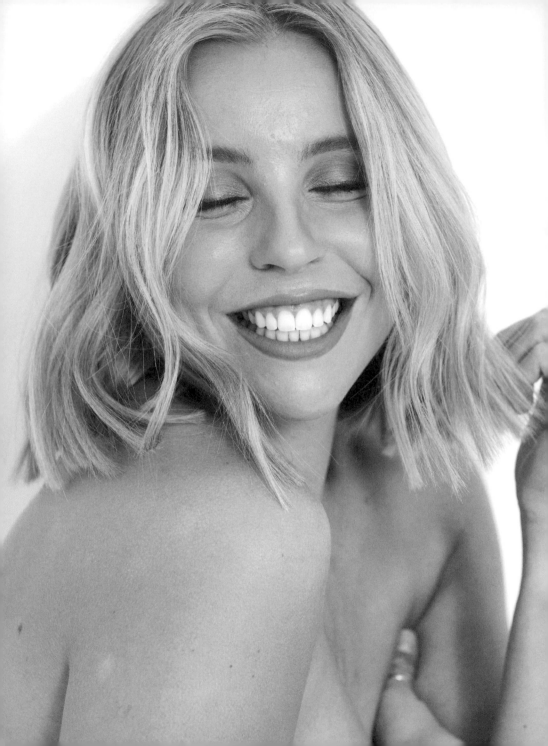

permanent solution while seeing different dermatologists. I was open to trying anything – I booked myself a series of LED light-therapy sessions, I cut out dairy, sugar and fat, I used all the topical creams available. I used to have evenings before bed where I'd squeeze one of them until I'd got out all of the gunk. Then I'd try so hard to resist having a go at the others, but then spend up to an hour attacking my face until it was bleeding and scarred.

Now, when I watch my red-carpet interviews back from this time, all I can focus on is my poor skin. Under the lights, the spots looked like they were bulging out of my face. I stopped presenting, turned down jobs, I really struggled to see friends, I cancelled dates last minute … it took me to a dark place and I felt plagued by these strangers taking over my face.

Watching Henry go into the same battle, fighting on the front line of acne, made me relive it all. Seeing him hiding his face under hoodies and hats, calling himself a 'spotty mess' and cancelling things so he could stay at home. We thought Brontë had escaped it all and was one of the three Kings to be blessed with forever perfect skin. But at 22 years old, she was recruited to join the war. We've all supported each other through it and it's affected us in different ways, but thankfully we've come out the other side, with some badass scarring.

Each year 3.4 million GP appointments are made concerning acne, so you are not alone, even if you feel like you are. If you've struggled or you are currently struggling with acne, **I feel you, I hear you. It is not forever.** When you've fought something for so long, it's hard to believe there's a way out. There will be something out there that can help you.

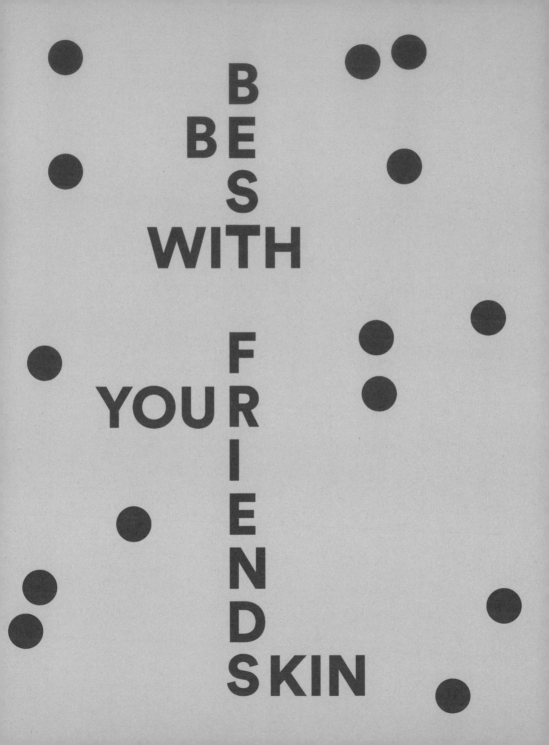

We're finally best friends, my skin and I. We fall out still, but I treat it with so much more respect now. There are days when I'll kindly ask the spots to fuck off from my face, especially in the 10 days leading up to my period. But ... I've found what works for me and my skin – it's nothing extreme, just a consistent daily routine.

Try a clay mask (my fave is Exuviance).

Wrap your fingers in tissue and gently press down on the base of the spot head. If it doesn't pop after two squeezes, leave it to do its thang.

Wash your face straight after sweating or if you can't, use Clinisept, which is anti-bacterial ... and try to not play with your face.

Use a natural cloth, like a cotton muslin (you can get three for £10 online), to take off your cleanser – your hands can't remove all the dirt and the cloth will gently exfoliate.

Use speakerphone or put on some headphones.

Those magnifying mirrors that make you see every teeny tiny little thing on your face ... just stay away from them. They're bullies.

If you find products that work for you, use them consistently, day and night. I would just use anything I could find that was in my cupboard because I didn't know what was working and what wasn't.

I found someone who genuinely cares and wanted to help me. I have a skin fairy godmother called Pam, a clinical aesthetician, and I went to her when I was desperate for help with angry and painful acne.

HERE ARE PAM'S PEARLS OF WISDOM:

Wear sunscreen everyday (factor 30 or 50 if you can), even when it's cloudy. UVA is out daily and penetrates beyond cloud and glass, directly into your dermal layers.

If you wear hats regularly, make sure you keep them clean. They harbour sweat and bacteria and can be the reason your head gets congested. If you have a fringe, or long hair, try to sleep with your hair off your face and change your pillow cases every four to five nights — especially in the summer, when it's hot.

Always cleanse with a gentle cleanser and never just splash it off with water. Use a flannel. When you splash, make-up, pollution, sweat and sebum will not be fully removed. This change alone can take someone from a few spots to no spots.

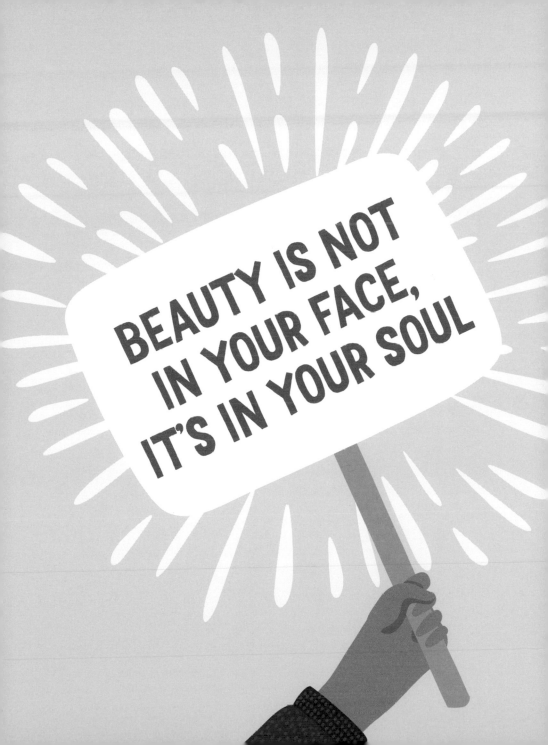

Me and my periods

Oh periods, how wonderfully magical you are, how powerfully painful you can be. You intruded on my life at 12 years old, but you still fascinate me every bleed. I am in constant awe of my body around my period – the biology of it all still amazes me. Also, why isn't it called the womenstrual cycle ...?

At nearly 27, I'm still a little caught off guard every month. It's like 'Bam, hey, remember me? I'm just going to be shedding my lining for the next few days, give me some time to do my job, will you? Love, Uterus'! I've felt a little out of tune with my cycle since coming off the pill a few years ago, but we're getting there. After losing my period through undereating and over-dieting, all in the name of a bikini competition (more about this later), I now look forward to getting mine. I am in no way an expert on this, but I just love talking about periods.

Looking back at my teen years, I find it funny that we didn't rally round, as girls, to support each other. When I got my first period, all I can remember is the feeling of the unknown. Everyone thought periods were gross, messy and an excuse to get out of everything. As if being on your period wasn't difficult enough, the humiliation at school piled on top of it all made it an extra-embarrassing time of the month. Tampons were treated like toys for boys – they loaded them up, pulled the trigger and fired them across the classrooms.

Code Red
Time of the month
'On'
Lady time
The 'blob' (my least favourite)
Mother Nature
Having the painters in
(or, as Mat says, the builders)
Shark week oo ha ha

NO THANK YOU, EUPHEMISMS ...
WE'LL GLORIFY THE WORD PERIOD.

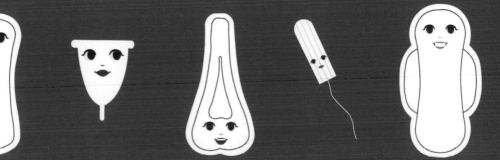

Pads felt like nappies and I would always stick them too far forward on my pants, which made me look like I had a big bulky vagina! Mumma taught me how to insert my first ever tampon safely. I had one foot on the toilet seat, jelly stuff around the cardboard applicator, and a seized-up body from crying. I absolutely hated the feeling of an alien object going inside me, a string hanging down outside of me.

MY TOP 3 'BLOODY HELL!' MOMENTS

I Waking up in a warzone three weeks into a new relationship with a boy who'd never had a girlfriend before. I'd bled through his bed sheets, onto the mattress … and somehow it was on the back of **his** leg.

II You know that magic trick where a napkin turns into a whole stream of napkins tied together? Well, that's what it felt like when I pulled out a tampon, then felt another string hanging down. I'd spent the whole day in pain, convinced I had appendicitis, but there I was, totally unaware I had 'doubled up'.

III Bleeding through white jeans on a date in the cinema. When the film finished and the lights came up I looked down **horrified** at my newly tie-dyed trousers and speed-waddled to the toilet. My jacket became an impromptu wrap-around skirt until I got home.

It's only been in the last three years that I've explored new period frontiers – there's so much more choice than when I was growing up.

Now, my favourite weapon is the cup; second favourite: period-proof pants. My cup and I have had a very intimate but all-round positive relationship. There have been quite a few 'Oh my God, it's stuck so far up me I swear it's touching my lungs and it's never coming out!' screams from the bathroom. My fingers have had to search so far up, desperately trying to catch hold of the teeny tiny rubber tail, yanking while trying to push it out with my ever-so-strong pelvic floor that was simultaneously gripping onto it.

The cup-of-the-moon (as Mathew calls it) and I had a breakthrough a few months later, when I realised I hadn't quite mastered the technique (I was shoving it a bit too far up) ... so we're now friends. If you've never used one or seen one before, I described it to Bee once as an Action Man-sized toilet plunger. It's a pretty marvellous invention, one that I wish I'd known about when I was younger.

Sometimes I still get caught out and end up doing the layer-up-a-load-of-tissue-and-stack-it-in-your-knickers-which-are-already-ruined-to-make-a-barricade trick. Imagine if there was a period-pant graveyard for all the knickers we've ruined: RIP (Rest In Pants), thank you for being there for us, sorry we weren't very prepared to save you.

As I write this, we are confirming the date of the wedding and I'm actually trying to work it around my period. With my cycle changing length every time, it's quite hard to predict, but I'm doing everything I can to make sure I'm not on my period because of the pain. Genuinely not wildly bothered about the blood and white dress combo, more so the way I feel and the lack of energy I have. So I'm just going to have little words with my uterus, praying for her to listen, in the run-up to the wedding.

Periods are something we should all be speaking **loudly** and **proudly** about. We're using our upstairs lips to talk about what's going on in our downstairs lips. We are taking back ownership of our periods.

A real-life 'flow' chart

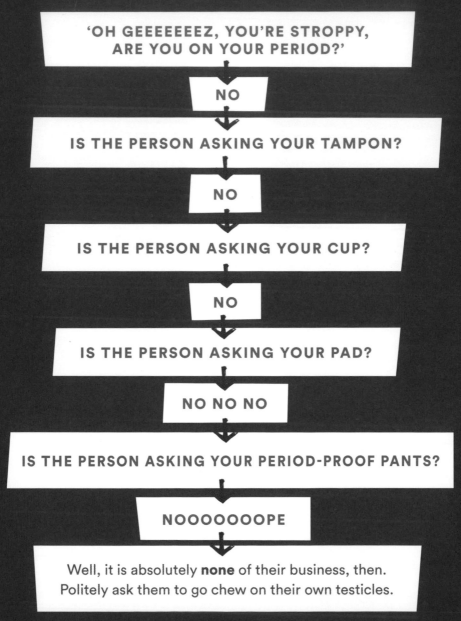

'OH GEEEEEEEZ, YOU'RE STROPPY, ARE YOU ON YOUR PERIOD?'

NO

IS THE PERSON ASKING YOUR TAMPON?

NO

IS THE PERSON ASKING YOUR CUP?

NO

IS THE PERSON ASKING YOUR PAD?

NO NO NO

IS THE PERSON ASKING YOUR PERIOD-PROOF PANTS?

NOOOOOOOPE

Well, it is absolutely **none** of their business, then. Politely ask them to go chew on their own testicles.

THE PAIN ... OH THE PAIN

The way I try to explain it to Mat is that I've invited two sumo wrestlers into my body. They've made themselves at home in my tummy and are tussling, punching, flooring and throwing each other around inside me. All in a 65-degree sauna before air-con was invented.

There is so much to learn about periods and why we get The Pain.

★ Period pains are most likely caused by an excess of prostaglandins – the compounds released from the lining of the uterus as it prepares to shed.

★ Prostaglandins help our uterus contract and relax, but pain can happen if our uterus contracts strongly, as it reduces blood flow and oxygen supply.

★ We typically feel our cramps in the lead-up to our period (because of the reason above), but sometimes we can experience pain mid-cycle, during ovulation, too (I get ovulation headaches, the kind of throb-throb-throbbing that delightfully ruins your day).

Please remember to give your body that extra time to do it's thang – take it as a reminder to slowwwww down and reeeejuvenate.

Me and my contraception

I lost my virginity a week before my sixteenth birthday – I couldn't quite hold off another seven days! I'd been with my boyfriend bang on a year and it felt like the right time.

The fumble pre-business. The tangle of gangly limbs. The squeaky single bed. The post-sex-bleeding-on-his-white-sheets. All while *Austin Powers* is blaring out in the background ... the soundtrack to my introduction to sex.

It wasn't quite the first-time experience I'd imagined in my head. No one gives you a map to follow; you have to navigate your way through it all yourself. You learn what you don't want and, equally, what feels **good** as you grow. You also realise the importance of contraception and, like period protection, that there's something that will work for you.

My brilliantly non-judgemental and understanding mum took me to go and get the contraceptive pill. I sat in the waiting room, anticipating the ever-so-slightly-awkward 'Francesca, are you currently sexually active?' chat with my GP who had seen me grow up. It felt totally different to the victory stories being gossiped about around school of those who had got to fourth and final base.

Back then, the majority of my girlfriends were on the pill – it was 'cool' to be on it; it showed you were having sex. At the time, it was seen as the easiest, simplest form of contraception. I had one friend

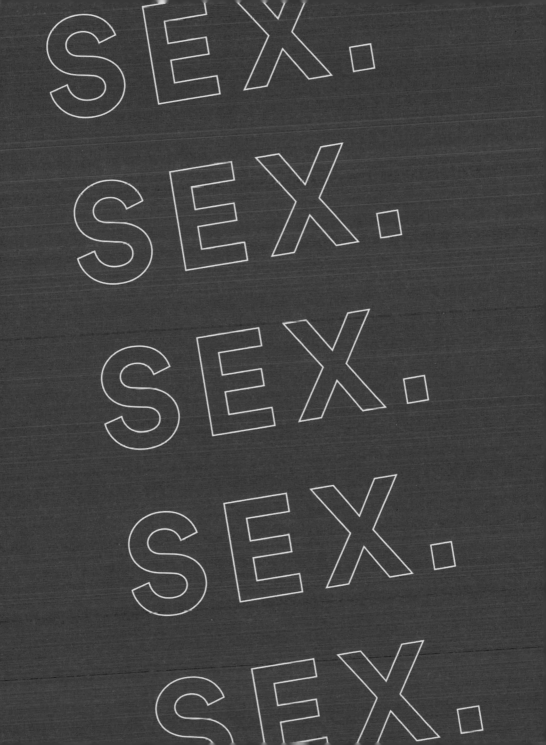

who had chosen the implant: it looked like a slug had buried itself in her arm and she played with it, moving it about … that totally ruled that out for me. And condoms? Boys used them as ammo, filling them up with water and throwing them at the girls in summer lunchtime breaks at school. My 16-year-old self thought they looked funny, they smelled funny and they hurt my fu(a)nny.

I was on the pill for just under a decade, but it wasn't until opening up online about some of the health issues I was having that I realised it could be causing a problem. I think social media has helped us all, as women, talk more openly about issues like hormones, contraception and everything that comes with it. After talking about my acne and how a few doctors advised me to try different pills to clear my skin, I found so many people were going through the same thing.

For me, I felt like the pill was making it even worse and my heart episodes were happening more regularly (my heart rate goes from 140 to 240-ish in less than 5 seconds … this is how I lost my hearing, but I'll talk about this later), which one doctor told me could be caused by the hormones in my pill. So, at 24, I decided I was done with poppin' it every day. I was ready to come off and start understanding my body naturally, without the added hormones.

I thought it was going to be a case of 'Boom, everything's back to how it was pre-pill, here's your period and a whole lot of your natural hormones, you're welcome, love Body.' But no.

It took 12 months to have any sort of bleed ... and even then it was a one-day period with all the symptoms that the pill had masked. I was crippled with pain, my hormones were **wild** – I just wanted to wrap myself in my duvet like a burrito, hide myself and my erupted skin from the world and eat my way through an entire supermarket chocolate aisle. After that it took another five months to have a two-day bleed, with my womb feeling like it was being ripped out. I almost considered going back on the pill just to dull the pain, but I promised myself I would listen to my body.

I was gripped by an overwhelming fear that I wasn't 'working' properly. I was convinced something was wrong. I took 10 pregnancy tests in a month (all negative) because I just couldn't understand why I wasn't on my period. So instead of self-diagnosing, I went to my doctor. I think I had a very unrealistic view of my periods, going back to how they were when I was 12. They reassured me it wasn't completely unusual – my body was just rebalancing after an eight-year supply of hormone.

When people ask me if we're 'trying' because I've come off, I say, 'I am, Mat's not,' and as much as I joke about it, I'm being deadly serious! I want to be a mummy more than anything in the whole entire world (hopefully I will be a fur baby mumma by the time you read this!). I've wanted a baby since I was four, convinced my sister was **my** baby! I genuinely think about it every single day. I can't walk past a baby without wishing it was mine; if there's one near me, my full, undivided attention is on the tiny bean! I have friends who have never felt that maternal desire – and that is absolutely normal, too. One of them said she'd never, ever wanted a baby; she'd always considered herself a good auntie but never saw herself having children of her own. She's now a glorious mumma, after fearing it the whole nine months of pregnancy. Whenever she's doubting herself or feeling like she's not good enough, I'll be screaming down the phone, 'You pushed a human out of your vagina, you are an actual superwoman ... you can do **anything**.'

Mat really wants children ... he absolutely loves them and I know he'll be a phenomenal father. But, he wanted to be married first – he's traditional and I totally appreciate and respect that. We're also very aware that it might not be possible; we've seen our friends either not able to have children or going through the trauma of miscarriages. This is, unfortunately, very common, and I think it's so important we talk about how hard it is for both the women and their partners. I know we live in a world with so many other options to explore, which is incredible, so I will find a way to be a mummy.

So for now, I'm tracking my period, for awareness but to also take back control of my cycle (and so I can pin Mat down the few days leading up to ovulation ... kinda joking – I'm not an animal, I promise). I trained to be a doula last year, which is someone who provides support for pregnant women before, during and after their birth. While I was learning and going through the course, I felt like I'd found **my** thing. It honestly makes me tear up even writing this. I get more fulfilment and joy out of being a part of a woman's journey to motherhood than any job or career I've ever done. It is the most empowering experience and I am even more in love with the human body after seeing what it's capable of. I'm incredibly grateful that I get to be part of life's most precious moments – the birth of a child and the birth of a mother.

Let's talk about sex, baby

Sex is the creation of life. Sex is why we are **all** here (or as my dad likes to think, it was the sharing of the same flannel while holding hands with Mum that made all three of us).

I really, truly love sex – it can be spectacular – but I wouldn't describe my sex drive as super-high, even now I'm with Mat, who I absolutely adore. I think I have more wild sex dreams than *doing* the actual thing. And as I've grown up, I've really discovered what I want in bed. I love that deep connection; I crave that feeling of skin on skin, taking me out of real life. Some weeks – the **mega** weeks – we'll have sex five or six times (ha, like two weeks a year!) ... but other weeks, we'll have absolutely none. We're both guilty – as I'm sure a lot of people are – of pulling out the 'I'm exhausted' card ... Sometimes good sleep wins over good sex.

I genuinely think there's so much pressure on us all to be:

Having sex
Having MORE sex
Having wild, experimental sex

I mean, I'm all up for contorting myself into a pretzel and snapping my hamstring getting into a level 6 position, but I'm not into whips 'n' shit. I'm more M&M's than S&M. Incredible if you are (come teach me), but I'm okay with being fairly plain, vanilla or just ordinary. Especially with underwear ... I never, ever got the whole sexy underwear thing. Mum still laughs at my £2 tooth-floss G-strings with holes in them and non-matching bras. The most experimental place we have sex is on the sofa in the living room ... and even then it's basically like doing it on a mini bed. I do have an orgasm prescription, though. Not a rule. A prescription. Because they're basically medicine to me – they make me feel so damn good. I won't stop until I've finished, whether that's making love to Mat or to myself.

Sex and love are both pretty exposing; they take courage and courage is vulnerability. I mean, in what other situation in life are you getting completely naked (apart from forgetting your socks) and fumbling around with another human?! Maybe naked Twister ... but I haven't played that for a while. I always used to think there was a correlation between sex and loving your partner. I thought the more sex you were having, the more you loved your partner and vice versa, but now I'm with Mat I've realised that is absolutely not the case with me personally. In fact, it has nothing to do with how much I love him; it's actually more to do with how I'm feeling in my body.

If I'm feeling confident and comfortable in my skin, I'll be at the top of my sex-game, but if I'm struggling with self-doubt and body-shaming **myself**, I'll whack on some chunky pyjamas and turn over to sleep. Sex or making love is different for all of us, it feels different for all of us, and it changes throughout our lives. Try new things and if it feels sweet do more of it. But if you're very happy with how you're doing it/not doing it, there's absolutely no need to change it up. I might not have the porn-star gene in me but I've got my own tricks and I'm good with that.

TURN ME ON

Be best friends with your contraception

What contraception do you use, if you use any? Let's take this opportunity to have a think about what you're using, what it does for you and the last time you checked in on yourself. Get your notebook out.

MY CONTRACEPTION:
pill [ ] condoms [ ] implant [ ] coil [ ] patch [ ] other [✓]

I've ~~been~~ *Not* been on it for: *2 years*.

Using it ma~~ke~~s me feel: *Out of control.*

(If you feel like it's controlling you and how you feel daily, maybe it's time to explore other options with a professional's advice/guidance.)

My last break from it was: months ago [ ] years ago [ ] never [ ]
I last went to the docs for a discussion about my contraception.............. days/weeks/months/years ago
(If it's over a year ago, book that appointment in now.)

Remember the mum from *Mean Girls*: 'Do you guys need anything? Some snacks? A condom?' Well, I'm **always** up for snacks … and maybe a condom, but there are so many other options. It's just about how you find the right one for **you.**

★ **Do** listen to your body. You know yourself better than anyone. Some methods might not agree with you.

★ **Do** your own research – there are some brilliantly informative and scientifically sound websites, like HelloClue.com, the NHS UK site and the Family Planning Association's Sexwise.

★ **Do** trust your GP – they can give you honest advice about what's available and how it works.

★ **You do not** have to copy your friends. We're all different and this isn't a decision to make on the basis of 'Well, Teresa *hated* her coil, it ripped out her flaps when the doc removed it …'

★ **You do not** have to let a man march you to go and get the morning-after pill if you don't want to. It is **your** body. You have the choice.

★ **You do not** have to be embarrassed. I'm pretty sure your GP has heard **everything**.

★ And **don't** use the pull-out/withdrawal method if you don't want to get pregnant. It's unreliable, it's messy and no one wants to clean up the aftermath …

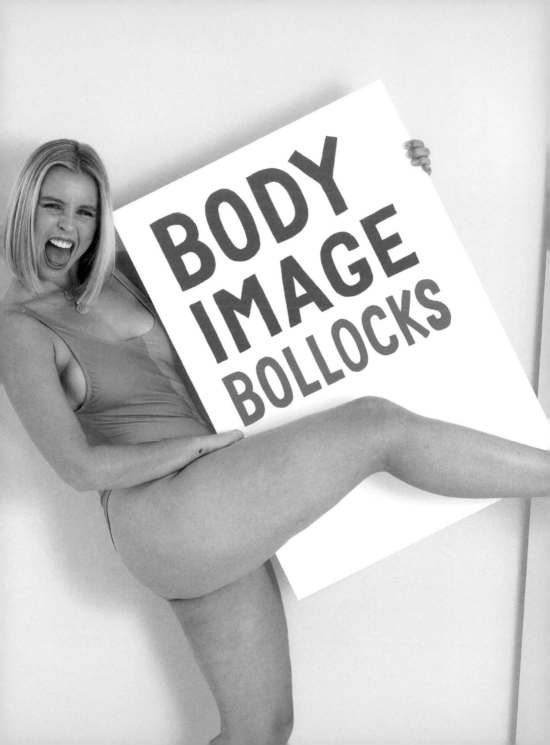

My Body and I

We have been on one hell of a ~~journey~~ EXPEDITION – we're finally best friends and I appreciate it more than ever.

To me, body confidence ultimately comes down to how I think and feel about my body **and** other people's, regardless of how it compares to any 'ideal'. Positive body image for me is not solely about how my body **looks** – it's about how I talk about my body and how I look after it.

Every day my appreciation deepens and I am forever fascinated by what our bodies **can** do. It's unapologetically celebrating the everyday things that feel like **magic**. Like the cut on my finger that heals two days later; the tingly feelings I get when I'm with Mat; it's putting my hand on my chest and feeling my heart beating, my lungs breathing for me and keeping me alive; it's watching my friends' bodies grow babies ... We are all capable of so much more than we believe.

It's taken me years of experiences, joy, grief, pain, extremes to think like this. I used to think confidence would come from all the added extra layers – the hair extensions, the immaculately polished acrylic nails, the 'skin-perfecting' make-up, the 'cellulite-busting' roller ... I subscribed to an ethos that I now call 'Body Image Bollocks'.

Bollocks to body ideals

I've always been a tall gal. At 13, I'd shot past Mum and Dad and towered over my friends at 5 foot 10 – in school photos you can see my head poking above everyone else's in the back row. I was the 'boy' in all partner dances in ballet. I was dedicated goalkeeper in netball. I quickly started to become aware of how much 'more' of me there was compared to my friends. I felt different and it was the first time I'd felt shame related to my body. I would round my shoulders and try to make myself their height – which did absolutely no favours for my posture! My friends were busy borrowing each other's clothes, but I couldn't even fit my baby toe into any of them. When I forgot my PE kit, I could only fit into the boys' kit left in the lost-property bin. My first ever boyfriend, at 12 years old, was a shorter kid nicknamed 'Munchkin', so it didn't take long for the whole of the school to label us 'Mop and Bucket' …

We've all been surrounded by images on the news, in magazines, on TV and now on social media of how a woman 'should' look. The so-called ideal, the 'perfect' woman. All these different sources embedded themselves deeply in my busy-growing-up brain. It had a huuuuuge effect on my sense of self-worth – I used to think that looking good was a strength, a power.

While I was digesting my way through being a teenager, I was being fed so many conflicting messages and images about womanhood and I felt like I needed to be **better** before I had the chance to even be **myself**. There was a constant hum of negativity in my brain, a voice making so much noise that I couldn't turn it off. I let my mind torment my body – my thoughts were the bullies, my body was the victim.

Before Instagram, I was an avid magazine reader. I would always stack them up for a long train or plane journey. There was a regular slot in my favourite mag laying out a female celebrity's 'food diary for the week'. Their average daily food consumption went a little something like this:

★ **BREAKFAST**
A doll-sized bowl of chopped papaya with a squeeze of lime and kiwi.

★ **LUNCH**
Two rice cakes, low-fat hummus and shredded carrot.

★ **MID-AFTERNOON SNACK**
A big-toe-sized portion of almonds after sucking on a green-tea bag.

★ **DINNER**
Half a tin of tuna on a bed of sad-looking lettuce and one tomato.

★ **DESSERT**
A fruity herbal tea and the remainder of the kiwi they didn't eat for breakfast.

That's what I eat in one sitting and I **still** feel hungry. But back then, it knitted itself into my subconscious, eating up all the healthy information Mumma had fed me. It made me want to look like the celebrity. It made me want to see if **I** could eat that little. It was a challenge, and I loved a challenge.

Difference. The only thing we all have in common

With social media in everyone's pockets, we're engulfed by perfect images that add to this mild brainwashing. No matter how confident you feel in your body, you can still fall into the trap of questioning whether you should be 'prettier', 'smaller', 'more tanned', 'blonder' – the persistent reminder that you can, and <u>should</u>, always look **better** just confirms your self-destructive thoughts.

The happiness thief is good mates with the comparison snake. It slithers in and wraps itself around you; it is poisonous. Now, whenever I catch myself even thinking, 'I wish I had her smooth, peachy, undimply bottom' while looking at a workout video on the 'gram, I remember how unique my dimply, squishy, lop-sided bottom is. How wonderful it is in its own way and that no matter how many crab-walky-bum-burny squats I do, it will probably never look like hers.

The **Our Outer Orbit** chapter (see page 203) is where I go in nuts-deep about social media. But I think it's important to recognise that it's only in the last few years we've had people openly and honestly talking about their bodies. I've come to a liberating place of love and acceptance for my body. I unsubscribed from looking 'better' but I am proud to say my body and I are more resilient than ever. I might not be able to chuck a 90kg barbell over my head, but our relationship is mighty strong.

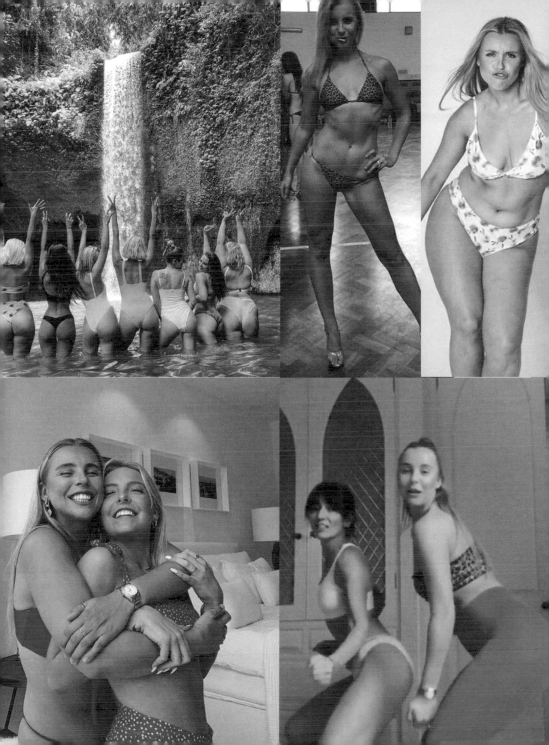

Going to battle with my body

From 16 to 23, I put my poor body through a pretty rigorous time. I was constantly told that my body needed to change. I was too big to model. Too big when I stepped on stage at 9 per cent body fat. Too big to be a dancer.

So I listened and made myself smaller and smaller and smaller ... I shrunk myself to prove to everyone I could be the size **they** wanted me to be. Just like the barcode on a packet of popcorn that shows its price when it's scanned – that's how I saw myself. I valued myself on my packaging. Not the delicious popcorn, not what was inside of me. My body, my outer layer, my 'shell'.

The slow-burning catalyst to it all came from a modelling agency, who'd scouted me at 17 years old. They brought me into their offices for headshots, sat me down in front of a queue of girls half my size, and told me they would only take me on if I lost 2 stone – **2 stone**. Feeling a cocktail of hurt, anger and fire, I replied, 'Oh good, so you don't want me then, you want someone completely different.' I walked out with a mighty urge to show them I was going to get work without changing myself! I wanted to break the norm and make a stand for future women who were being told they weren't good enough.

I went to a few castings – off my own back – still adamant I wasn't going to change my body for a modelling agency. But every single one broke off a little piece of my confidence. One girl I met in the queue for another life-sucking, image-bashing casting turned to me and asked if I could hold her place while she went to the toilet. She came back looking washed-out and fragile. She was a stranger to me but a sister in that queue. Without even thinking, I gave her a cuddle. I didn't say anything, I just held her brittle body and she started shaking in tears on my shoulder. She told me she was so desperate to get this job, she'd left a chicken breast out for

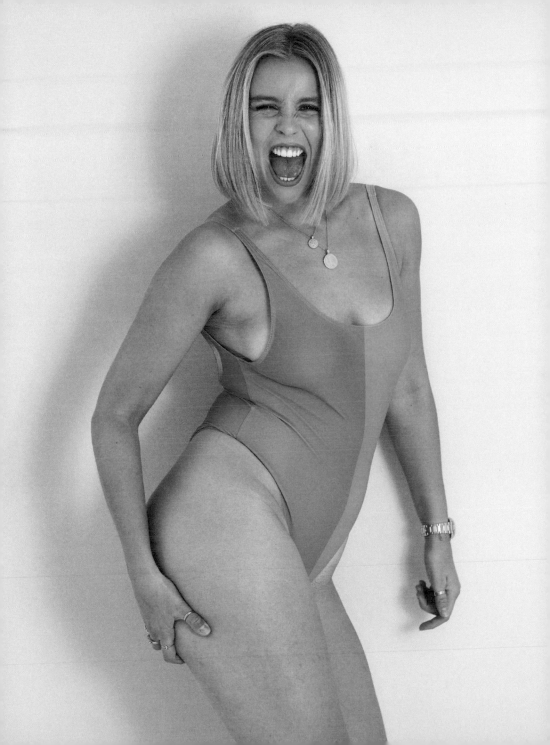

four days past its sell-by date, cooked it the day before and eaten it – deliberately, to make herself ill. She hadn't stopped being sick, all night and all morning. I felt sick **for** her; she was a prisoner to the industry. I never saw her again but every time I went to a modelling job, all I could think about was her.

I never went to an extreme like that, but I started eating less, losing weight rapidly. I started lying to myself, my mum and everyone around me. I knew I needed help but I didn't want to be rescued. I didn't want to hear other people's advice on my body, on my eating, on their own experiences with overexercising. I would come home after long days of drinking coffee and not eating properly, but would tell Mum I'd already had dinner. I'd wake up the next morning with my tummy rumble as my alarm. The diet culture had ensnared me and I bowed down to it like it was a religious cult.

I stopped eating after 6 p.m. I stopped eating anything that contained fat. I wouldn't touch anything that wasn't a green vegetable or quinoa. I ate side portions of kale while everyone was eating pizza. I took bites out of bananas then squished the rest into the bin. Friends would order me food when we were out, but I wouldn't eat it, just mix it around in the hope they'd think some had been eaten.

In six months, I went from people commenting, 'You look incredible, you've really lost some weight, haven't you?' (**side note**: as much as I'm sure people were trying to compliment me, it's just reinforcing body-image messages. Which isn't helpful, as people see it as a positive, so therefore strive to meet that compliment's expectations. I'll talk more about reframing compliments later on …) to, 'You look really unwell. Your ribs are sticking out. You've gone too far now and you don't look like the Chessie I love.' I thrived on being told I was 'too skinny'. All I cared about was being the smallest version of myself I possibly could be.

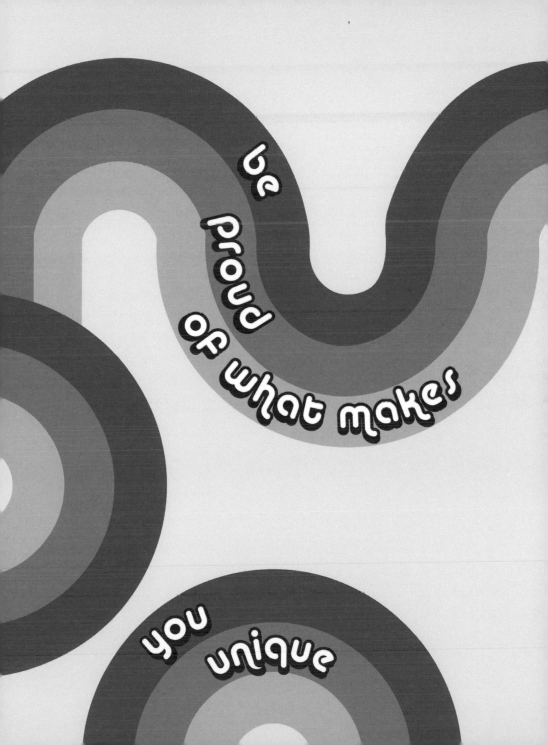

Using and losing my voice

At the time, I was also dealing with medical issues, which pretty much changed my future. I had struggled with my voice from the age of 12, losing it for weeks at a time. Cameras were stuck down my nose and throat to find a rather chunky cyst on my vocal cords. Imagine a bunion, protruding from the side of your foot. Well, that was what was going on in my vocal folds … gross.

Musical theatre was my life and I'd been accepted on a course at a school that specialised in performing. After my first operation was unsuccessful, I was booked in for a second go. My teeny tiny vocal cords had taken a massive dissection to remove a cyst. (FYI – it's not safe to google images of 'vocal cord X-rays' in public … When I got my scan back, I thought they'd done it the wrong end, as they look like two labia folds. I said to Mum, 'Are you sure that's not my vagina?!') I was told I would have to learn how to talk properly again, with two weeks of complete silence to heal after my ops. I was also warned after both that I wouldn't be able to sing for a year. The musical theatre school wrote to me saying they wouldn't be able to risk training me and couldn't take responsibility if any permanent damage occurred, so my place was taken away, a week before I was meant to start. I was 19 and I felt like my future had been ripped apart and thrown on a fire.

In true King style, when a door slams closed in my face, I go somewhere else where the doors are different, welcoming and open. After 24 hours of crying and working out what to do if I couldn't do what I had dedicated my whole life to – presenting, dancing, singing and acting – I was on the computer, googling 'unexpected, unplanned gap year'. I found Camp America, something I thought only existed in the movies. Ten weeks of teaching kids dance in Maine sounded ideal.

Do you have tea and biscuits with the Queen?

Always … though it gets a bit dull every Tuesday sitting in Buckingham Palace with the corgis piled up on my lap. Just playing; I'm unfortunately not best friends with Her Majesty – this is the greeting I received from my 'bunk kids' when they heard my 'queen accent' and where my nickname 'Biscuit' came from.

I landed in Maine, extremely underweight and dangerously hungry, after six months of religiously restricting my food and working out relentlessly for hours on end. All I could think about was food, watching everyone eating and thinking I was the only one who knew the calorie content of half a banana. The first two weeks, I was terrified of the buffet food; I had demonised everything that wasn't a green vegetable. I would make it look like I was too busy to eat at mealtimes, instead going around the table, making sure all of the kids were eating.

One evening, two weeks in, one of the girls shouted from the other end of the table, 'Biscuit, all you do at mealtimes is drink water and eat broccoli.' They had started picking up on my unhealthy ways. That comment was exactly what I needed. 'I can't be setting a bad example for these very impressionable young girls, I need to stop,' I thought.

That night my mum called. Brontë had shown her a photo of me that I'd uploaded on Facebook. Looking back now, I cannot believe how tiny I was – I'm unrecognisable. She made it pretty clear that they were all really worried about me. The following evening, as part of a competition between the camp counsellors, I ate 34 Oreos … Thirty. Four. Oreos. My poor, poor digestive system! I hadn't even looked at chocolate, let alone eaten it, in six months.

Even though it was pretty extravagant, at the time it felt like a gutsy move and it quickly reignited the love I'd previously had for food. When I landed back in the UK, my family were so relieved. My friends told me I looked 'wholesome', 'well-fed' and 'healthy'! I thought I was 'fixed' and I told myself I'd never put my body through starvation again … but it was just a temporary camouflage.

Teeny weeny bikini competeeni

In 2015, I walked on stage in a gold barely-visible-to-the-human-eye bikini (that cost me £650). I was the colour of a mahogany table after being smothered in six layers of fake tan (which cost another £150). I was taking part in a bikini competition. I had trained my ass off and eaten broccoli for breakfast for 18 weeks – for something lasting a total of 40 seconds.

Why did you do it, Chess?! **Oh** why, oh why did I?! Honestly, at the start, I saw it as a science experiment; I wanted to test what my body could do, what I was capable of. It then became more about the willpower and proving to myself and others I could do it. Now I look back and see how unnatural it was for my body – you could've picked me up with a pair of tweezers and put me in your pocket … but at the time I really felt like I was doing it healthfully.

The hardest bit was psychologically coming back to normality post-comp. For the first week, I genuinely didn't go a minute without eating. I couldn't stop. The weight piled on and I stopped training completely – rebelling. As if that wasn't hard enough, my coach had asked for feedback from the judges a few days after the competition … They said I was too big and I was carrying too much weight for my group. That stung. Real bad. How dare they? One delightful comment from Mr Anonymous was, 'You look like you've eaten your friend. No wonder you didn't win.' Really helpful, buddy, thank you for your concern. Go pluck out your pubes and eat them.

It felt like a massive kick in the vag and everything I did for those 18 long, hard weeks felt like an absolute waste. But I was soon to get a message from my body that I'd gone too far.

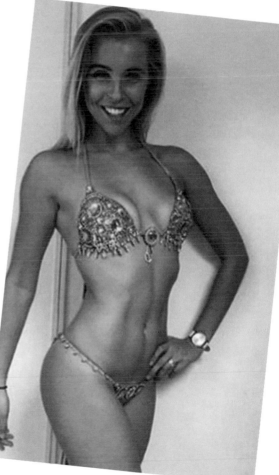

Hear me out

I was 23 when I lost 70 per cent of my hearing in my right ear and gained tinnitus (a constant high-pitched ringing). After multiple tests, brain scans and doctors' diagnoses, they have said now it was most likely a mini stroke.

It happened during a boxing class. Most people's reactions are either, 'Wow, what happened to the other person?' or, 'How hard was the punch?' I kinda wish it was a knock-out story, but in all truth, it was just me and a boxing bag. It was my second class of the day and it was only 10 a.m. My nana had passed away suddenly a month before, I'd split up with Hamish, which was all a bit messy, and the only way I could deal with the grief was by working out, **hard**. I was absolutely hammering my poor body, masking the emotional pain with physical pain.

Ten minutes in, I was already exhausted, but my mind was distracted, so I carried on. My heart rate shot up from 160 to 240 in just five seconds as I looked, blurry-eyed, into my watch for my heart rate. Suddenly, I woke up on the cold floor, my body gyrating with every fast beat. I thought I was having a heart attack or a fit. Crawling out of the class, I could only hear this loud high-pitched ringing sound and the quiet muffled noise of people around me. Lying on my back outside the class, people were towering over me. I couldn't hear what they were saying; I could just see their mouths moving.

They turned me onto my side and covered me in cold towels. With deep breaths, and a lot of convincing myself I wasn't about to die, 20 minutes later my heart rate came down to a steady pace. As I stood up for the first time, my left ear popped. But my right one stayed blocked (and has done ever since).

I felt totally disoriented but needed to get home. I tried to explain to my parents what had happened, but I scrambled for words, unable to string a sentence together. Mum spent the whole weekend with me trying to create a completely Zen space with yoga, early nights, baths, googling every magic ear trick we could find. We all thought my hearing would eventually come back, like on an aeroplane when you feel like your head is in a fish bowl when you land and then the next day you wake up and can hear again. But it didn't.

The grief of losing nana was a huge stress on my body with all of the crying, not sleeping or eating well, and then I was pushing myself to my maximum, day in, day out. No wonder my body went to that extreme to tell me to stop. I wear a hearing aid when I'm presenting and I'm a pro at asking people to repeat things, but it still really affects me in some situations. I've had 12 episodes since losing my hearing where my heart rate has skyrocketed to 250bpm. It's extremely scary and wipes me out for the rest of the day. But, hopefully by the time you read this, I'll be post-operation. I've just been diagnosed with SVT and I have a hole in my heart. It feels incredible to have a clearer understanding of what's happening and I feel so supported under an incredible cardiologist – after 3 years, I've finally been heard. I'm having a 'LINQ' fitted, which is a device implanted under my skin near my heart. It will record my episodes for up to 3 years. Then they're going to go up through my groin to my heart (while I'm fully awake) to burn off a few extra electrodes up there and fill in the hole with a bit of plasticine.

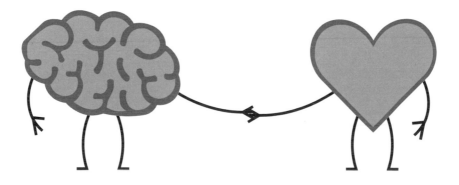

My body is my home for the rest of my life

It took me going through all of that trauma (and more) to find that eternal friendship with my body. It's not an A-to-B kinda thang; it's more like the **entire** alphabet, stopping at every letter along the way. It didn't just happen over a few days. I didn't buy a fast-track ticket to all the rides: I waited in the long seven-year queue. But it was all worth it.

One of my friends was really struggling with her image recently and I asked her to send me a message about her home and why it feels like her happy, safe place. She sent me a voice note saying how much she loved her bed where she sleeps, her table where she eats, her walls where she hangs all her memories. I listened to her listing off the things she loved. She didn't say, 'I hate …' once. When she'd finished, I replied, 'So why are you saying you despise your arms, your legs, your tummy? They are your body – your home for the rest of your life.'

No one knows your relationship with your body and what you've been through together unless they've lived inside your body **your whole lifetime**. We all have our own stories, chapters we've written and pages we've learnt from.

We still have moments, days when we fall out, my body and I. My old thought patterns start poking their heads up, like, 'Oh, hey, we're still here, remember us?' But I can recognise it, allow it and give myself a little pep talk.

The two things that have genuinely helped me the most – because they've actually worked long term – are:

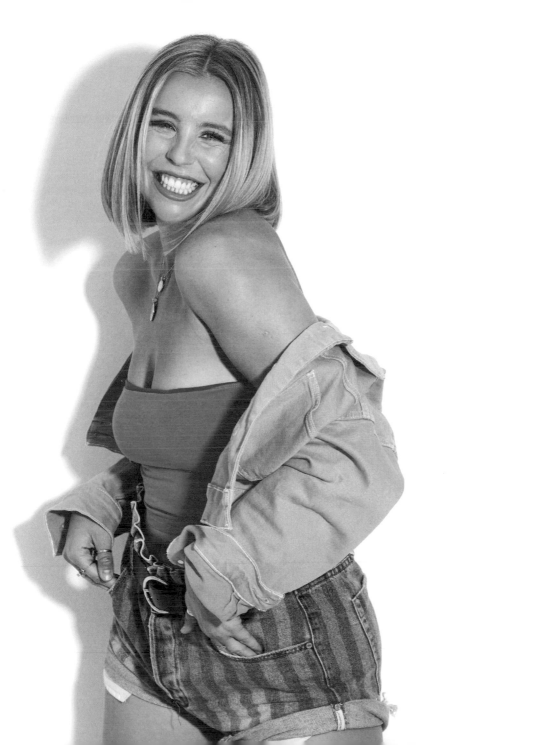

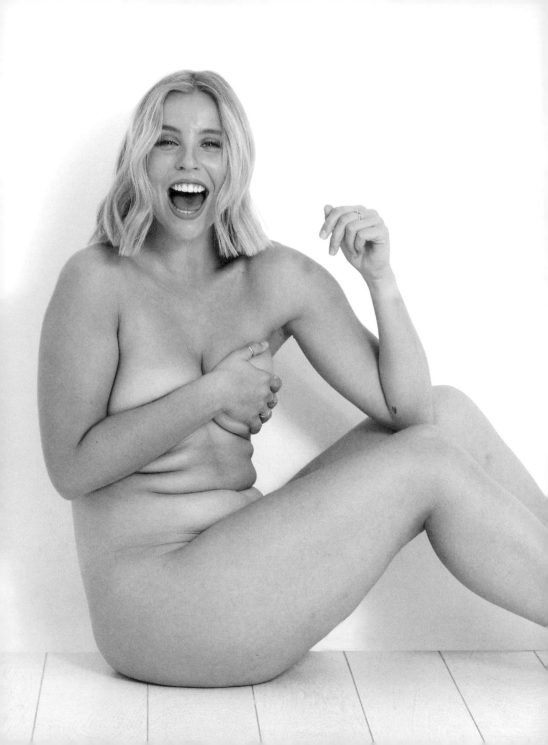

★ Speaking about my body in the way I speak about my best friends' bodies. I always ask myself, 'Would I let anyone tell me my thighs are too chunky and they look gross when I sit down?' **No**. 'Would I ever say that to anyone, a stranger, a best friend, my sister, my mum?' **No**. 'So why would you say it to yourself?' I cannot say it enough – I literally want to record it as your ringtone, set it as your alarm ... **Be your own best friend**.

★ Knowing my body and I are far more interesting than how we look. I love taking myself through a mini-biology lesson and really thinking about all of the hard work it's doing for me <u>right now</u>. There's a whole lotta work going on under your skin, so welcome to my academy of body-ology. Think about your eyes reading this book, think about your brain taking in all the words, think about the sounds around you and what your ears are hearing, think about your lungs breathing for you, think about everything your body has done for you since you popped out, up until this day.

I created the hashtag #DearBodyThankYou a few years ago, encouraging people to write a letter to their bodies. If I need to shift my headspace, I either read over one I've written or scribble down a new one. Let's do one together: write it down without any judgement in your little notebook of magic or in your notes on your phone.

Dear Body,

It was never, ever you that was the problem. It was me. Being a giant dildo to you.

I appreciate you and everything you do for me, thank you, thank you, thank you …

We can finally go away on holiday together, wear a bikini and make memories without me wanting to cover you up with a towel or a baggy T-shirt.

We can finally feed you all the yummy food you deserve without asking for the number of calories at a restaurant or throwing half of it in the bin.

We can finally go work out when we want to and work out as hard as we want to.

I can finally post photos of us without wanting to edit out every flaw. And I can finally stand up for us when people try to Photoshop you like they have done in the past. I can use our relationship and our experiences to help people feel less alone and alienated.

I wish I could go back to when you were your tiniest, during the time in our life when I left you so empty. I wish I could cuddle you and tell you you're not just on this planet to lose weight and have a permanent residency in the gym. You were worth so much more than your weight back then. You had so much more to give the world without me limiting you.

You put up with me trying to change you in every way, but when I pushed you to your extreme, you warned me I'd gone too far. Thank you. I know it took me a while to listen to you but I really needed it. I don't believe in failure, I believe we went through our difficulties and I've learnt from those fuck-ups, and they've shaped us.

I'm sorry strangers' comments about you have affected the way I think about you; they've got me when I'm feeling vulnerable. It's not us, though, it's them, it's society's warped views. I promise I will continue to talk to you with kindness, no matter what they say about us.

All the times everyone else told us we were too big, I believed them, before I believed in us. But I've learnt through working together that anyone who judges us is unfortunately unhappy in themselves and they need to blow our candle out in order for theirs to burn brighter.

You're hopefully the future home to my babies; my children and I cannot wait for us to go through that magical process together.

All of our happiest times together are absolutely nothing to do with how we look – they are with our friends and our family. All the things I used to hate about us are now the things I celebrate. You are bloody magical and I am SO thankful for you. I promise to protect you. I promise to take care of you for the rest of our life.

Love me, your best friend,

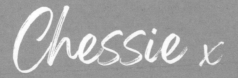

Chessie x

YOU ARE NOT USELESS

YOU ARE NOT WORTHLESS

YOU ARE NOT THE CLOTHES SIZE
YOU WEAR

YOU ARE NOT THE WIDTH
OF YOUR WAIST

YOU ARE NOT DEFINED BY THE
ATTENTION YOU GET FROM MEN

YOU DO NOT NEED TO CHANGE
ANYTHING

YOU DO NOT EXIST TO PLEASE OTHERS
WITH YOUR APPEARANCE

YOU ARE THE STRENGTH
OF YOUR AMBITIONS

YOU ARE THE POWER BEHIND YOUR CHOICES

YOU ARE THE DREAMS YOU DREAM

YOU ARE THE CHALLENGES YOU'VE FACED

YOU ARE THE RISKS YOU'VE TAKEN

YOU ARE THE BOOKS YOU'VE READ

YOU ARE THE FEELINGS YOU FEEL

YOU ARE THE PLACES YOU HAVE
TRAVELLED TO

YOU ARE THE MEMORIES YOU'VE MADE

YOU ARE THE PODCASTS YOU LISTEN TO

YOU ARE THE SONGS YOU SING

YOU ARE THE THINGS YOU BELIEVE IN

YOU ARE THE LOVE YOU FEEL

YOU ARE THE OWNER OF YOUR BODY,
YOUR BEST FRIEND

You are pheno-wo-menal!

Before we zoom out to Our Solar Support System, I just want you to take this moment to absorb everything from this section.

Know that you can always come back to the bits that really spoke to you, the letter you wrote to your body or simply the words you connected with. And know that you don't **have** to be in love with your body, you don't **have** to be best friends with your body. You don't **have** to do **anything** that doesn't feel good for you and your body.

Hating our bodies shouldn't be the norm, just because you hear it from everyone around you. It's not your fault; it's not your body that is the problem. Wherever you are reading this, remember: you have lived and survived your entire life until this second. The hate, the heartbreak, the trauma, the grief, the loss, the wonderful moments, the painful moments … but look at you, you're here. Things are shifting, changing, we're seeing diversity, we're shouting about inclusivity and challenging opinions, shattering expectations. I really hope that right now there's someone on the front cover of a magazine, billboard or social-media campaign you can relate to.

Next time you catch yourself speaking negatively to yourself, ask yourself, 'what good could I be doing with my time right now?' Don't stop believing in yourself, forgiving yourself and reminding yourself you are unstoppable. Put this book down, put your left hand into your right and give it a little squeeze. You're a team. Look after each other. It's just you two, for the rest of your lives. The most powerful team.

GET
OUT
OF
YOUR
OWN
DAMN
WAY.

I'll say it again . . . .

GET
OUT
OF
YOUR
OWN
DAMN
WAY.

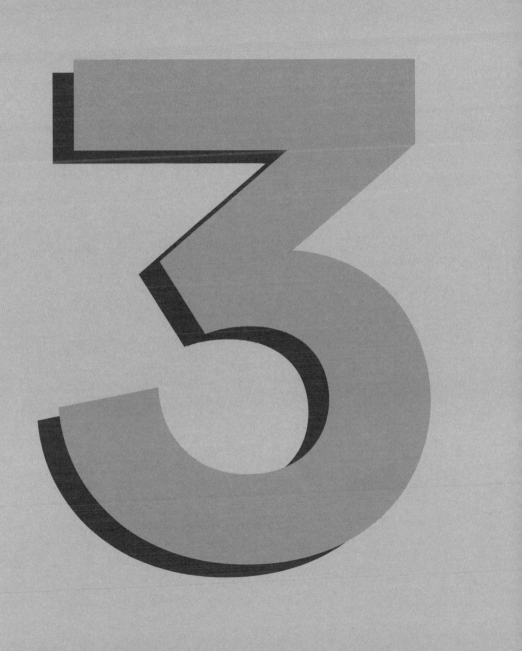

OUR SOLAR SUPPORT SYSTEM

THE ONES WHO MAKE YOU FEEL UNDERSTOOD, REALLY GOOD AND PART OF A SISTERHOOD

Together

There's this restaurant in London that serves DIY doughnuts for dessert (yes, we're absolutely going there together – message me an evening and I'm all yours).

You're given a plate of mini squidgy balls of deliciousness and four syringes full of different jams to inject into the middle. Our lives are like the doughnuts – damn tasty in their own right – but our favourite humans are the syringes, filling our lives with all their different flavours, enriching our doughnuts, making our lives so much more scrumdidddlyumcious.

My life has been (and still is) upgraded to first class by the special people closest to me – my extraordinary family, my marvellous Mathew, my supercalifragilisticexpialidocious friends and the champions in my work troupe. Our stories are different, our experiences are different, we're all different humans … but that is what makes life so bloody wonderful. It's not just me who knows there is true healing power in loving and being loved, there are doctors out there actually prescribing intimacy.

So let's dedicate this section to all the people who make us feel gooey, full of sunshine and FIERCELY indestructible. The humans who remind us we are never alone in life. Together, we'll explore how we can cherish these relationships and when to know a relationship isn't making us feel guuud.

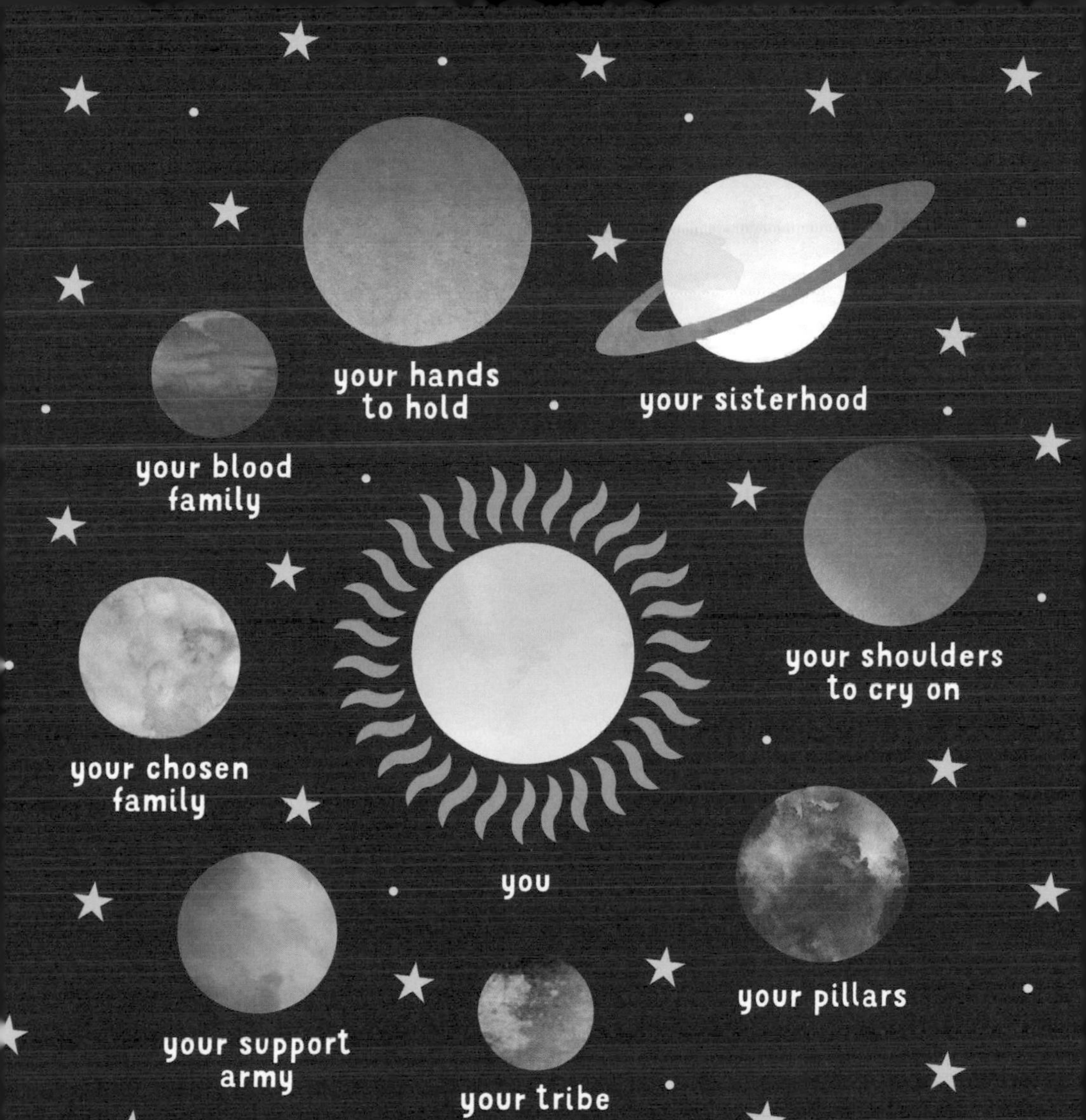

your hands
to hold

your sisterhood

your blood
family

your shoulders
to cry on

your chosen
family

you

your pillars

your support
army

your tribe

YOUR SOLAR SUPPORT
SYSTEM

LOMA LINDA
IN CALIFORNIA

THE NICOYA
PENINSULA
IN COSTA RICA

There are five
regions in the
world where
journalist and
author Dan
Buettner claims
people live longer,
HEALTHIER lives
than average:

SARDINIA
IN ITALY

ICARIA
IN GREECE

OKINAWA
IN JAPAN

The lifestyles of these 'BLUE ZONES' captivate me. But one thing that really stands out is the research into their super-duper-strong communities. People have an incredible level of social engagement and they all look out for each other, whether that's their neighbours, sisters, brothers or their buddies.

Research shows loneliness damages our bodies – it's the equivalent to smoking 15 cigarettes a day and is nearly twice as harmful as obesity. (A US study found that lonely people had a 50 per cent increased risk of early death, compared with a 30 per cent risk for obese people.)

We all need our communities to thrive – and that doesn't mean you need a colossal list of friends – even just one or two people can boost your life. Believing in yourself is a superpower, but when others believe in you it can magnify your life.

Friends

Friendship is so precious to me and I treasure every single one of my relationships – male and female. My friends are my extended family and, in each soul, I cherish their unique qualities – they unlock a different part of me. When I was younger, I was always that girl who woke up before everyone at sleepovers, too excited to sleep because we were spending the day together. After-school play dates with my friends were the highlight of my week. I absolutely loved my friends before I even KNEW what love really was.

I think it's more important than ever to truly appreciate and nurture our relationships. With social media, we live in a world that's trading in a new currency – the currency of likes and followers. In the past it has been money, but that's not always been visible – your boss doesn't have an 'I earn £75,000 a year plus bonus' sign on her desk. Whereas followers are on show for everyone to see, and it's so easy to think people's followers are a mirror of their popularity. I believe friends give my life true meaning: they enrich me daily and they are all invaluable. I love who I am around my friends, especially the feminine energy – it's unbeatable.

You can look at someone with 2.6 million followers on Instagram and think they have all the friends in the world. That could be the case – there are people who have strong online and offline networks. But there are also people with huge followings who feel lonely, unhappy and lost without real-life connections. That's what I call a friendship deficiency. There's no pill to take for it; the only supplement is to surround yourself with real-life, good human beings. Not just for the SOS moments when something goes wrong, but daily. I know people on social media who have given more attention to their online audience than their actual friends. Further down the line, they have realised their lives lack substance and, more importantly, have a deficiency in physical face-to-face interaction – which has led to social anxiety and generated a feeling of dejection.

I find it ironic that 'social' media takes away a piece of real-life socialising. Instagram, Twitter, Facebook and Snapchat all simulate the feeling of keeping in touch with your friends by liking their photos or commenting with a love-heart emoji. But that to me is surface-level communication. I thrive on deep conversation – asking questions, listening, really finding out how that person is, how they're feeling; nurturing friendships is a constant thing. Sometimes, I think we need reminding that no amount of likes on Instagram can ever substitute a real-life squeezy hug from your best friend.

But sometimes that's not possible, and we're so lucky with technology and phones nowadays that we can carry our friends around with us in our pockets, all over the world. I try to keep connected to my friends who I can't see all the time by doing one of these:

Let your friends know you're there for them ...

Start a WhatsApp group with a few of your closest friends.

Send little quotes to each other in the morning.

Have a rule that you see each other at least once every month. Choose a date and stick to it and make it phone-free.

Send silly photos/videos.

Ask everyone what they're proud of after a long day.

Be open and honest when you feel like shit.

Allow them to rally round.

Open up and ask for help.

Send voice notes to each other.

FaceTime each other.

Send little presents to their work.

Handwrite a card or a letter.

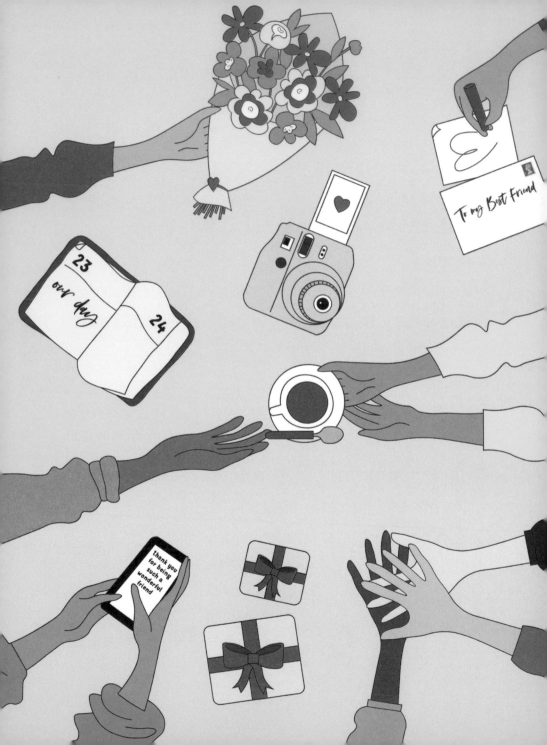

THE POWER OF FEMALE FRIENDSHIPS

There have been centuries' worth of female friendships. Our great-great grandmas had a girl gang; they're all probably up there together, squeezing each other's spots, taking each other home after a big night in heaven's one and only club, and coming on their periods at the same time because their cycles have synced.

Some of the best moments in my whole entire life have been with my best friends. They are my greatest loves. I've grown up with a sister, my ultimate BF, where there has been absolutely no jealousy or bitchiness from either of us. From day one we have been obsessed with each other. It's an indescribable love and has taught me so much about friendship.

But the past few years have been revolutionary in my female friendships – I've really refined, understood and strengthened my circle. I can now confidently say I KNOW who's in my **forever sisterhood**. You know that feeling when you find those friends who just get you: you understand each other, you trust each other, you thrive off each other and you cherish each other. There's no judgement, you feel safe when you're together and when you're apart. I adore Mat, I adore my parents, I love my Hen, but there is nothing like quality time with my best friends, my SISTERS, my future bridesmaids, my children's future godmummies.

My close circle is the backbone of my solar support system and it's an eclectic mix of energy, love and celebration. I am forever thankful for the superwomen that I'm lucky enough to call my friends. I've learnt that you can't rely on one person to do everything, to support you in every way. They all add to my life in different ways and as Beyoncé once sang, they're irreplaceable. They know who they are.

So, let's celebrate all your different kinds of friends and honour them. You can share this list with the people you love, or just keep it to yourself as a reminder of all the **heroic humans** in your life.

Big up your besties, your golden friendships, and check in on all of them today.

MY CALM AND COMPOSED CONFIDANTE
Thank you, _Twinnie_, for your calmness, delicate and gentle nature and _for your never-ending_

support. Love you ridiculous silly amounts,

together we are unstoppable and we understand

each other on such a deep level.

MY ROCKET-FUEL FRIEND
Thank you, _Angel Skye/Banana Girl_ for your infectious, divine energy, your effervescence, your passion and

your ability to make me smile no matter how

many miles there are in between us and for

doubling up as a removals woman all the times

I've moved house, without me even asking.

MY HERITAGE HOME GAL

Thank you, *Miiiige.*, for putting up with me since day one, for knowing everything about me, your loyalty and *our archive of indescribable memories.*

MY S-EXPERT SISTER

Thank you *Georgie*, for your invaluable advice, your extensive penis and vagina knowledge and *Your fountain of fanny-tastic fables.*

You've got to allow your friends to teach you, to take you out of your comfort zones and make you say yes to things you wouldn't normally do.

171

THE EVOLUTION OF FRIENDSHIPS

I like to think of our whole entire existence as one long-running box set – the memories you make with your humans make up the 'episodes'. Just like your favourite series, there are some eps you want to watch over and over again on repeat, but there are some you want to skip or remove from downloads. Just like our emotions, hormones and bodies change as we get older – our relationships also develop, acclimatise and shift throughout life. I think it's really important to recognise that relationships can be compli-fucking-cated and **that is okay**. Just like everything in our lives, friendships evolve.

If you're reading this and thinking, 'I still haven't found my female tribe, my solar support system doesn't exist, **you are not alone**. It absolutely does not mean you're any less of a person or you need to go searching for and auditioning friends. It could mean that these people are already in your life. You might just need to spend more time or open up and be more vulnerable with them. Or it could mean you've got to be honest with yourself and prune your friendship group.

I've never been one to argue, and I don't thrive on confrontation, but as I've spoken about in the section on honesty in Chapter 1 (see pages 42–9), some of my friendships have developed through truthful conversations. I always go by how a friend is making me (and the people around me) feel. I believe it's all about the energy a person puts out. Now I don't like to categorise or put people in boxes … but recognising how you are before, during and after seeing a person is a good way to understand if they're adding to your life:

RADIATOR

SOMEONE WHO GIVES OUT WARMTH,
LOVE AND SUPPORT. THEY FEED OFF
POSITIVITY, YOU FEED OFF THEIR
POSITIVITY.

VAMPIRE

SOMEONE WHO SUCKS ALL OF YOUR ENERGY
AND ZAPS YOUR HAPPINESS. YOU LEAVE THEM
FEELING DEFLATED, UNINSPIRED AND DRAINED.
THEY FEED OFF NEGATIVITY.

STAY CLOSE TO THE PEOPLE WHO FEEL LIKE

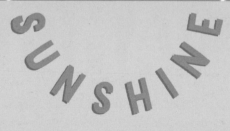

SUNSHINE

but be there for the people who are stuck in their
own storm, hold an umbrella over them to stop
the rain and guide them through the darkness

Just like most of us, I've had experience with vampires guzzling and slurping my happiness in the past. But the older I get, the more I realise that these people are sometimes the ones who need the most help and support. If you feel like you can't give that to them, guide them to a support line or someone who is qualified to give advice. Always go back to a place of empathy if you can and be gentle. If they felt like a vampire when you last saw them, it doesn't mean they're a bad person – they might just need help. Over the years, the clearer my true friendship group gets, the more it fills with radiators. It's one big cosy party huddled around a fire toasting marshmallows – the people at the party make me feel warm, comforted and loved. That's because I've learnt who makes me the happiest, and for me the most important thing: who makes me feel like I can just be myself. The most raw form of myself.

If I was struggling with anyone at school, if I was being left out or talked about behind my back, Mum would always point out that at school you don't get to pick the people you're put with. 'Once you get older, you start choosing the people you want to spend time with and those you want to give your energy to.' (Oh, you're so wise, Scrumma!) At the time I couldn't really comprehend all of that. When you're a teenager, school feels like it'll never end, and you'll be behind a desk with mountains of exams until you're 92. But now I realise she was so right.

I know how much friendship break-ups sting – they can feel like a real, physical injury. Just know your worth and if you're starting to see a vampire in a friend, trust your gut. Maybe you're just not complementing each other as friends right now because one of you is going through change or self-development. You might be able to come back to grow the friendship – it doesn't have to be the very end.

Rather than seeing it as losing friends, I see it as part of the evolution: solidifying your network of true friends as you grow old. I look back and realise I didn't lose anyone; I just gained a better understanding of what I want, what I really, really want (a zig-a-zig-ah!).

HOW TO BREAK UP WITH A FRIEND (WITHOUT HURTING EITHER OF YOU)

Just like all relationships, you have to start out a friendship with an open heart, to allow those initial connections and build up trust through vulnerability. When it clicks, it really clicks and you feel invincible together. I know how it goes: you make future plans, get dates in the diary and the next thing you know, you've spent every single day for the last three months together, you've shared secret stories, you're glued to each other; you're now well and truly best friends forever …

BUT THEN, ONE OR MORE OF THE FOLLOWING THINGS START TO HAPPEN:

Dates become exhausting; all they want to do is gossip and talk negatively about other people.

You walk away questioning whether they speak about you like that to their other friends.

She stops replying to your messages but carries on Instagram Story-ing and posting like you're non-existent.

There's a double-tick graveyard on your WhatsApp chat – all the message bubbles from you start piling up.

You start questioning things – yourself – looking back at texts and digging around for something you said.

You go the whole day checking your phone every minute, seeing her 'online', waiting for the 'typing' … but nothing.

You type out a message on your notes, going back and editing until you have a final version … you send it, reading it back for the 23rd time to make sure you've worded it right. She comes online straight away.

Her response is a kick in the boobies – she starts blaming you for things, lists out things she thinks you need to change – a word-vomit you weren't prepared for … wow. It knocks you flat on your back like Miley Cyrus coming in hot with her big old wrecking ball.

Your friendship has become a friend**shit**. You feel like your friend has just taken a big old dump on you and you're left with all the mess.

So. We need to protect ourselves and choose the healthiest decision for us. It's human instinct to be defensive but when you are your own best friend, you don't need to self-justify. You're self-assured, you **know** when it's a **'It's not me, it's you'** kind of sitch.

If this has happened more than once with the same friend and you feel like you've been let down multiple times, there might be more to it. It's so difficult when you've been through grief, loss or trauma together. I've had that bond, that emotional attachment to a person because we've felt pain together. You built a history with your friend. You built a future with your friend. You thought you knew them back to front, inside out. But let's go back to reminding ourselves; we never, ever know what someone is going through, even if they're our best friend. Once you start realising they might be struggling with something they haven't shared with you (or in some cases ANYONE), ease off the pressure you built up on yourself, and give them time.

Now, unless this person has done irrevocable, permanent harm or damage, there is the possibility to **recover** this friendship later on down the line. No one tells you how to break up with a friend; there aren't classes in this shit. But I've learnt from experience and want to share with you three ways to say ciao, adios, I'm done for now (thank you, Anne-Marie!).

177

1. GET IT ALL DOWN

I've found writing a letter to that person really, really helps. I have named and addressed it to them with no intention of sending it or them ever seeing it. It's therapeutic, getting it all down on paper. You can burn it, rip it up or keep it in a safe place. Let that shit go. Let that shit grow.

2. PREPARE WHAT YOU'RE GOING TO SAY

The reality is that some friendships do have to end. Recognise and respect that you have had some wonderful memories together but right now you can't give anything to the relationship. If you do it over the phone or in real life, have a list of bullet points that you know you want to say. You don't need a full script but having little prompts helps you in the heat of the moment.

3. FEELING = HEALING

Just because you're the one making the call, it doesn't mean you can't find this a difficult time, too – you have a meaningful history together. Speak to someone you trust, a family member or someone who isn't a mutual friend. Give them a logical lowdown of what's happened so you feel like you're supported throughout.

You're three steps down, so I'm going to bring you four steps up. Let's champion the value you give as a friend and recognise your unique personal quirks, which are not wrong but could be misinterpreted … I invite you to scribble down yours, too.

THINGS I'M PROUD TO SAY I OFFER AS A FRIEND

I have always been very affectionate. All of my friends say it's like hugging a boyfriend or their mum when they squeeze me. I love a cuddle, I love a hold of the hand, I love a stroke of the hair.

I always try to be supportive no matter how busy I am. I get so excited for my friends for both the small victories and the gigantic ones.

I like to think of myself as a 'safe space'. I am a very good listener — it all goes in and stays in. I remember conversations and the little-but-valuable details from months ago, sometimes even years.

I'm always 'available'. If a friend is in trouble, needs help or is struggling, I will be with them PDQ (pretty damn quick). Wherever I am in the world, I will find a way to be there for them.

THINGS THAT DON'T MAKE ME A 'BAD' FRIEND BUT WHICH I KNOW AND AM AWARE OF

I'm not good at feeling unappreciated. I love a thank-you and that's because I have been brought up to say it for even the smallest of things. I've just realised that some people don't see it as such a big thing; they might be thankful but they show it in different ways.

I sometimes feel like I know more about my friends than they know about me but that's because I don't allow myself to be heard sometimes. I tend to deflect questions about myself, but I know that's a huge part of building up a relationship. Mutual vulnerability. I'm getting there and starting to open up more.

I'm not great at knowing what I need and I don't like ever feeling I'm burdening people when I feel like steamy shit pie. Sometimes I think I can just deal with it all in my head, but my friends know me so well — they can tell when something is up.

You don't have to work on these things, they're all part of you. It's just being aware of how they can impact other people.

We are FAMILY – I got one sister and brother with me

Family might be traditionally defined as the people you are related to by blood, but to me it means so much more than that. Family can be a blend of partners' families, step- and half-siblings, step-parents, godparents, extended family, cousins, neighbours, childcare providers, babysitters – basically anyone who you can completely trust and rely on.

I never, ever take for granted how lucky I am to come from such a strong, well-built foundation. My parents, my sister and my brother are pure golden humans. The support of the four of them makes me feel invincible – as if I can do anything. A huge amount of my strength and confidence comes from knowing that even if I fail, they are there to patch me up.

I've learnt so much from my family of six humans.

'Treat your family like friends and your friends like family'

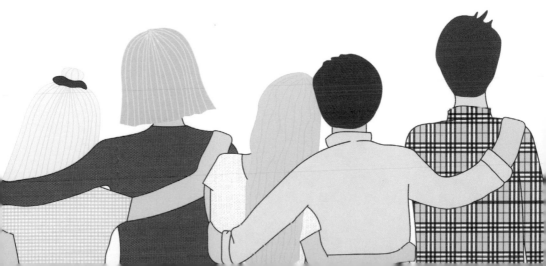

I GOT IT FROM MY SCRUMMA MUMMA

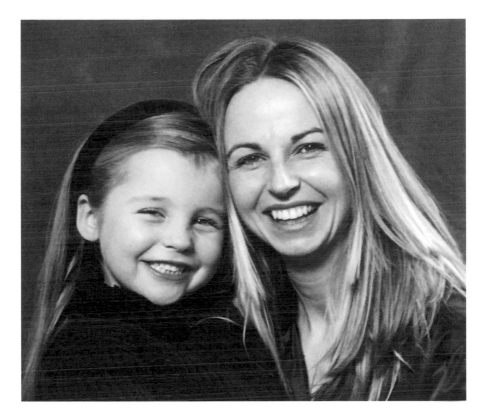

Mumma

Me Julie. Scrumma-mumma-doo-dah. An icon.

I have spoken about my mumma a lot already, but I could honestly write the whole book about her: her benevolence, her infectious energy and how she lay the foundations for us as children.

Even before she had me – before it was 'trendy' and there was even an awareness around needing to be healthy – she was interested in it all. She did her own research, then eight years ago she trained to be a yoga teacher. And in the last few years she has been studying for an evidence-based diploma in applied nutrition.

From the moment she stopped breast-feeding me to now, she has cooked delicious, nourishing meals from scratch and has installed a deep-rooted understanding of the importance of food. She'd fill our school lunches with healthy and tasty food: nuts, fruits, vegetables and hummus. As a result, Brontë, Henry and I grew up with our friends looking at our snacks like they were aliens!

As much as she encouraged us to make healthy choices, there were never any restrictions; she just wanted us to enjoy healthy foods and understand the benefits of them. We were never forced to eat anything and, equally, Mum never stopped us from eating anything. We had the freedom to make our own choices with an understanding from a young age of what to fuel ourselves with that would make us feel good.

I did rebel against her, as we all do when we're growing up – we all think we know better than our parents. But the older I get, the more I appreciate everything she taught us.

I will try everything to be the same loving, caring and informative mum to my children. If I don't quite live up to Mumma King's standards, at least they have their grandmother to run to! She'll be downward-dogging until she's 95 …

Bee

Brontë Bee, where do I even start?

After four years of being an only child, my parents asked me if I wanted to be a big sister, and I honestly couldn't have wished to hold that title any more than I did. I didn't choose Brontë to be my little sis, but I did choose her to be my best friend as soon as she popped out – best choice ever! I was four when I met my baby sis, and I've since watched her grow up from a teeny tiny bean to an absolute queen.

B has always encouraged me to take risks – she was the one who made me start up Instagram, sharing my presenting clips.

B has always been so supportive. There's never been any competition.

B makes me see things differently, from her younger eyes.

B knows me better than anyone else in the whole world.

B has taught me how you can be a warrior even while battling with being a worrier. I have learnt about her anxiety and how I can be there for her when she's struggling. She has taught me how overwhelming panic attacks are and what triggers them – how to calm her down but also respect how different we are when it comes to fear.

We have the strongest relationship. We have our own language and understand each other more than anyone – sometimes we will have conversations that our parents listen in to and they say they have no idea what we're saying!

We have each other forever + ever + ever + ever, no matter what.

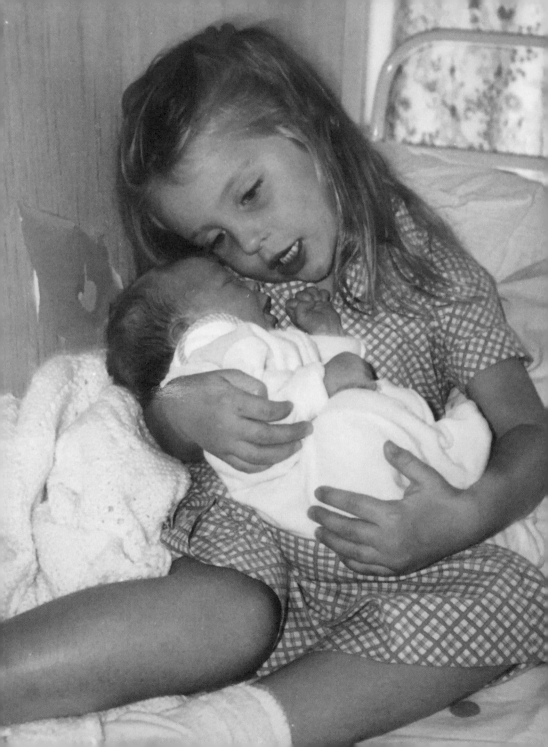

'OUR ROOTS
SAY WE'RE
SISTERS.
OUR HEARTS
SAY WE'RE
BEST
FRIENDS.'

Daddadadio

Who's the daddy? You the daddy. He has worked and still works incredibly hard, passing on that work ethic to all of us. He is forever humble, and says, 'There's a limit to the amount of credit a parent can take for the success of their children. Mum and I just gave you the building blocks.'

He has taught me to be fearless – he has taken risks all his life and spoken openly about them to all three of us.

Dad grew up surrounded by women. He has three sisters so he's always been super-understanding and empathic to Brontë and me. He met Mum just after his Dad passed away when he was 18 and they've been together since 1982. Mum waited nine whole years for him to propose, which Mat took on as a target to beat … 'Your dad's an icon, Chess. I've got to add a year to that. Ten years is a perfect amount of time to warm up that knee.' (Since writing this, Mr Carter has proved me/us all absolutely wrong, he knocked off six years' waiting time!)

Dad instilled in all three of us his love of music – there is never a meal without background songs, or a weekend without the sound of his Sunday-morning playlists. Stevie Wonder, Aretha Franklin and Frank Sinatra were the soundtracks to my childhood.

I cannot wait to be walked down the aisle with you by my side.

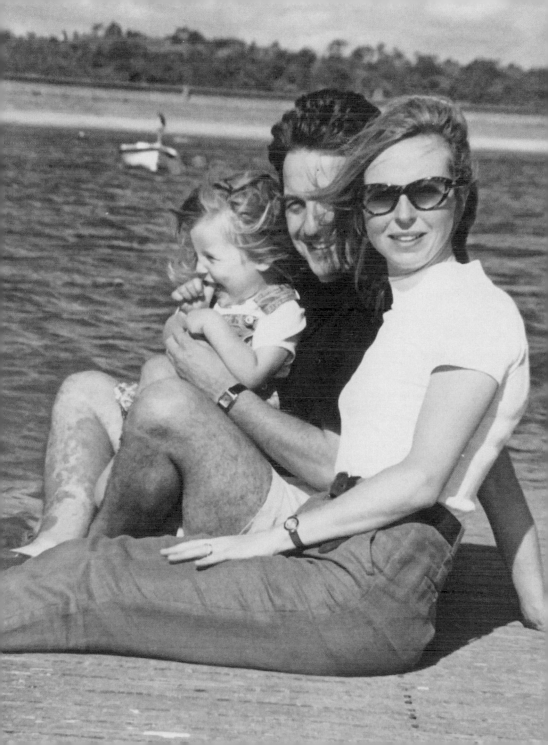

Henny Boy

I didn't fill out an application form to be a big sister a second time, and this time to a little brother. I had trained for three years with Brontë before H landed in the world. At seven years old, I'd had all the practice in changing nappies, holding floppy heads, after Mum had breastfed. I was a professional big sister, it was my favourite job title and I loved Henry a ridiculous amount from day one when I sat holding him in hospital like a trophy, showing him off to all the midwives.

At school – when I was going through puberty – I used to think, '**Oh please**, boys, you're fine, all you have to deal with is erections, your voice changing and your willy growing (or not).' Then I saw H

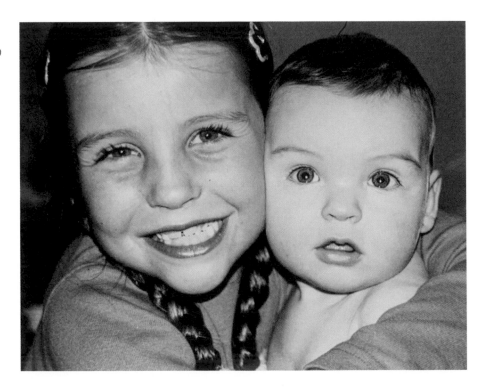

go through a lot of change, especially with his skin, where acne really knocked his confidence. There's just as much pressure for guys – to 'be strong', 'man up', 'grow some balls' ... all of which I believe should be removed from every human's vocabulary. Having both a brother and sister has taught me a huge amount, watching the different chapters in their books.

Hen is seven years younger and seven million inches taller than me so I can tuck under his arm and feel like his little sister! He is my daily source of entertainment and I honestly just adore his caring, patient and hilarious soul. Whenever I've thought, 'All boys are dicks. I'm done with men for the rest of my life' when I was struggling with relationships and dating, Henry and my dad have proved to me they're not.

'The greatest gift our parents gave to us was **each other**.'

Nana and Papa

Grandparents make the world a little kinder, a little slower, a little softer and a lot more special. Nana and Papa (my mum's parents) looked after me while Mum and Dad were working, so I spent a huge amount of time with them growing up. They taught us to be kind to everyone and to always tell the truth, Papa would say 'look me in the eye and tell me without fibbing' – my nose crinkles when I'm lying so I never got away with being dishonest.

They showed me life can be simple but still so wonderful. That forever and ever love exists – Nana and Papa were together for 59 years before Papa passed away on Nana's birthday. They taught me the magic in hand-writing letters, which I still love doing; they would write to each other when Papa was in the war, and back home Nana would ask the postman every day if he had a reply for her. They were so precious. I adored them and miss them a huuuge amount. Thinking

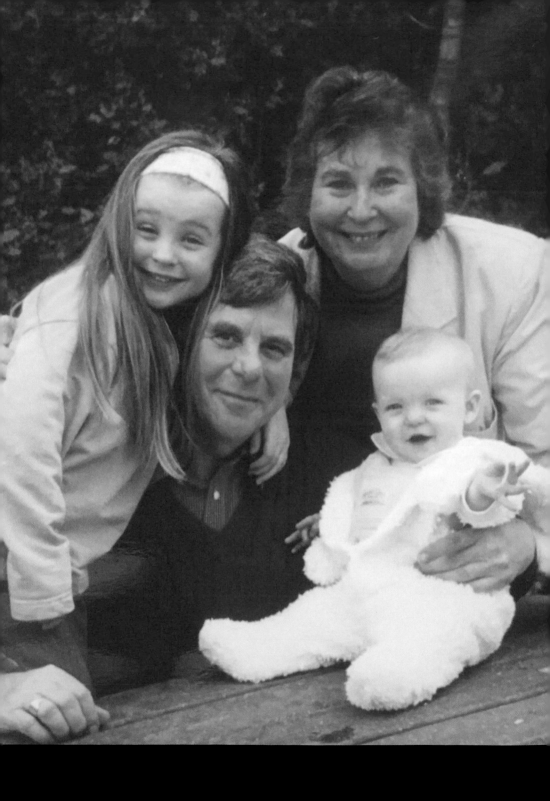

about them makes me excited to have my own grandchildren … might need to pop out a few children before that happens!

Nana passed away just before I started going out with Mat, in January 2017, I just wish he'd met them but I keep them alive by telling him stories about them. I try to remember them both for all the happy, healthy and special memories instead of picturing them how they were when I saw them last.

> **'Grief is really just love. It's all the love you want to give, but can't. All that unspent love gathers up in the corners of your eyes and in that hollow part of your heart. Grief is just love with no place to go.' JAMIE ANDERSON**

Family can be muddled, complex and chaotic. I appreciate how different all of our circumstances are and you may have read this section not being able to relate to any of it. I was honestly very wary to even write this chunk, as I didn't want it to look like the 'ideal' household. But there are broken parts in our broader family tree; it just wouldn't be fair for me to share these. Two of my best friends lost their dads in the same year, which was just unimaginable and tragic for them both and I felt like I went through the grief with them. I'm sending every ounce of love to you if have been through family loss; it really is an unexplainable suffering.

'Everyone has their own story; you don't know what chapter they're on or what pages they've turned.'

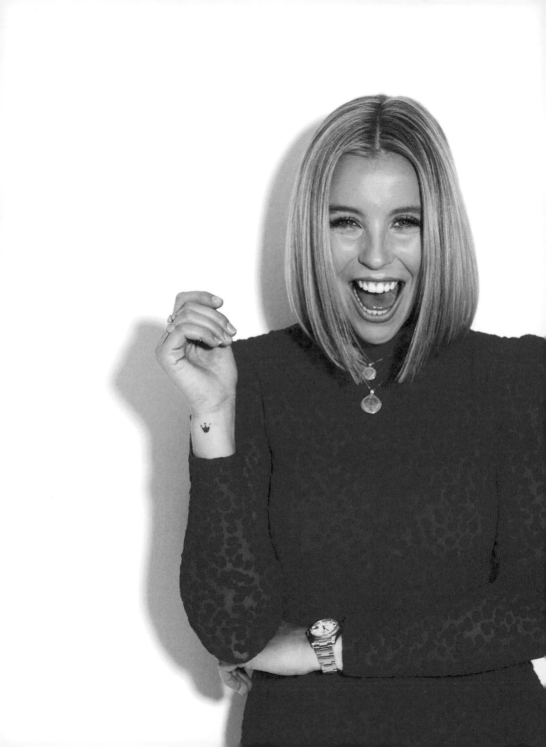

Wurk wurk WORK people

Working with women can be the epitome of empowering. You and Doris respect each other, you get shit done together, your desks are so close in the office you practically sit on each other's laps, you both fancy Tom from marketing, you leave each other little notes in secret code when you are separated for a minute, you share your drawer full of emergency period stash, you take turns in organising the office parties, sending Tom the first invite. Doris isn't just your work wife – she's practically your life wife.

I've read that it takes more than 200 hours with someone to develop that 'close friend' relationship. So it's not a surprise when you find that bond pretty rapidly with someone from work – you could be spending nine hours a day with them, five days a week. So in just under five weeks of Doris starting at your company, you could question how you ever lived without her. I have five Dorises in my team and I bloody adore them: Jen, Kat, Pip, Grace and Sean (Sinead). If I could, I would shrink them all down to pocket-sized versions of themselves so they're all with me wherever I go. There's also a very special, important human who deserves a strong mention: he's a Doris (but with balls, not boobies) who does all the behind-the-scenes stuff that no one realises goes on apart from him.

I've been in jobs with absolutely no Doris in sight and the office has felt like a very lonely place. I've been made to feel like the size of my baby toenail by bosses and I've witnessed office gossip rocket out of hand. It's only as I've grown up that I realise they all could've been going through hell at home outside of work ... or maybe they were just out to get me. They made me feel like I was useless, underappreciated, not good enough and that they were embarrassed to have me working for them.
I would lock myself in the toilet in tears and I'd come home from work every evening questioning what was wrong with me. I felt like I was the only one it was happening to, but now I'm older I know I wasn't alone.

You may not have colleagues but Doris could be your teachers, your mentors, your counsellors, your lecturers, your coaches, your team mates. The more we all lift each other up, cheer each other on and create an environment where we all want to work together (men, women and non-binary), the more we'll all thrive, achieve and grow.

You don't need to get on with every single person in the office, but if you are struggling with a work colleague or you're in a situation where you feel undervalued and it's affecting you, this may help: there is not one person on this planet who is entitled to treat you like shit. Please remember that and please talk to someone you can trust about it, outside of your work.

STAND UP FOR YOURSELF

What advice would you give your best friend if she were in your situation? Wait, who's your best friend? Did I hear you say I AM?! Yes, I'm a-talking 'bout you. Call a meeting and be honest with them. Flick back to pages 42–9 to give yourself an extra dose of bravery, and if you need back-up get someone more senior in the room with you. (If it's your bawsss that's the problem, get someone else from your team who can see what's going on.)

WE ARE ALL LOVEABLE

What a healthy relationship means to me

Supporting each other
Adding to each other's lives
Mutual respect
Honest and open communication
Spending one-on-one time together
Enjoying time without each other
Feeling safe in their company
Undeniable trust
Making each other laugh
Accepting one another's bad days
Having healthy boundaries
Inspiring and encouraging each other
Sharing decisions
Recognising when the other needs space
Listening to each other without judgement
Involving the other in your circle
Showing love and affection

WE ARE STRONGER TOGETHER

No matter what shape, size, history or story we have, we're all navigating our way through life. We're all still working it out as we go, but we can help each other along the way. Let's not allow people to pit us against each other – let's shift perceptions on female friendships and the beauty in them. Our voices are so much more powerful and loud if we all rally round and support each other.

Be your own best friend

Being your own best friend isn't about being your **only** friend; it's about honouring yourself and being proud to share yourself with others. It's about taking the advice you'd give to your best friend – and using it for yourself. You're putting love and energy into your tribe, but never forget to keep some back for yourself … I honestly believe the better you know yourself the better your other relationships will be.

This is a list, for you and your best friend (that's you), to help you realise you're not on your own. I've been through (still go through) every single one of the below and I wish I'd had someone to speak to about it and tell me I was not the only one, that it was all just a part of growing up and becoming who I am today.

MY BEST FRIEND AND I ARE TAKING TIME AWAY
TOGETHER TO REKINDLE – I DON'T KNOW
HOW LONG WE NEED, BUT WE'LL BE BACK SOON.

MY BEST FRIEND AND I ARE GOING FOR LUNCH
TODAY, WHEREVER WE WANT, JUST US.

MY BEST FRIEND AND I ARE STAYING IN BED
TO WATCH A FILM WE'VE WATCHED 23 TIMES
INSTEAD OF GOING OUT WITH EVERYONE.

MY BEST FRIEND AND I ARE OKAY WITH NOT
EVERYONE LIKING US; WE LIKE EACH OTHER.

MY BEST FRIEND AND I ARE GOING TO TRY
SOMETHING NEW – IT'S A RISK BUT WE'RE GOING
TO LEARN FROM IT.

MY BEST FRIEND AND I ARE REALISING WE'RE
NOT BEING TREATED RIGHT AT WORK AND IT'S
TIME WE STUCK UP FOR OURSELVES.

MY BEST FRIEND AND I ARE LATE FOR A MEETING
BECAUSE WE GOT OUT OF THE SHOWER, PUT ON
SOME MUSIC AND DANCED NAKED AROUND THE
HOUSE FOR AN HOUR.

MY BEST FRIEND AND I ARE PUTTING ON MAKE-UP,
DOING OUR HAIR, PUTTING ON HEELS AND WEARING
A BLAZING OUTFIT TONIGHT BECAUSE WE'RE
FEELING GUUUUD.

MY BEST FRIEND AND I ARE GETTING TO KNOW
EACH OTHER, DISCOVERING WHAT FEELS GOOD
DOWN THERE AND EXPLORING DIFFERENT WAYS
OF PLEASURING OURSELVES.

MY BEST FRIEND AND I ARE FEELING TITS-DEEP
IN SQUELCHY, SHITTY SELF-DOUBT TODAY AND
NO MOTIVATIONAL QUOTE IS GOING TO MAKE
US FEEL BETTER.

MY BEST FRIEND AND I AREN'T BEST FRIENDS
YET – WE'RE STILL WORKING THINGS OUT, BUT
WE'RE GETTING THERE.

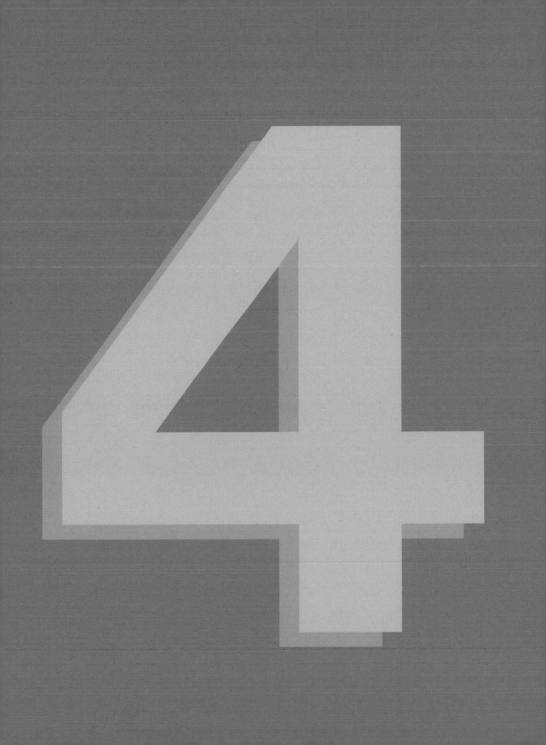

OUR OUTER ORBIT

STRANGERS,
DANGERS
AND GAME
CHANGERS

Our Outer Orbit

Imagine you're looking at a map on a screen. You start with the specific location – that's you. You zoom out and see the road you're on. You zoom out a bit more and see the town you're in. You zoom out even more and you see the country you're in. You keep zooming out and you're an astronaut in space – looking down at the big wild wonderful world and everything in it.

Well, this section, the final chapter, is all about that last zoom. We've peeled back all the layers – we've delved deep inside your yummy juicy bits, we've celebrated your bod and all the wonderful things it does for you, we've stepped out of ourselves and celebrated the people around us, and now it's time to unravel everything else going on in our outer orbit. Unsocial media, strangers and the noise.

I believe all women around the world are connected. We understand each other, and as I've been lucky enough to travel the world, I've seen how our similarities unite us all. The woman behind the counter in a foreign supermarket is a stranger to me, but I feel like I know just a little bit of her – we've both been through

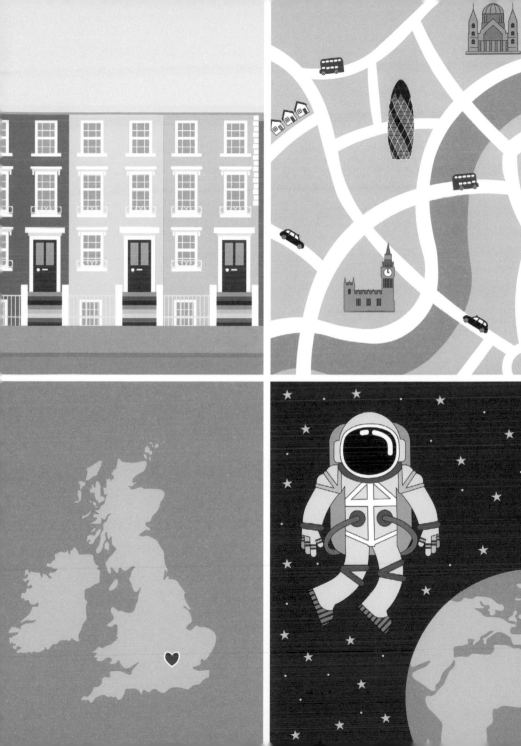

change, we've shared experiences, we are both dealing with the noise of the universe and the people in it. We've faced adversities, we've confronted judgement and criticism – all while trying to figure out who we are and what we want. Connecting with women is as effortless as holding a door open for a mumma with a pram; it's as simple as smiling at the girl who's sandwiched between two 7-foot men opposite you on the packed train; it's giving your elderly neighbour a hand with her shopping – no matter how dinky these gestures are, they can make a whole lotta difference.

Our great-grandmummas (and all of those who make up our DNA) didn't have the opportunities, the freedom, the ability to choose their futures like we have. I want to honour our history, continuing our great-great-great-grandmas' work and all the women who came before us.

But having modern-day freedoms doesn't mean that things are easy for us now – far from it. Society is always judging us as women. We're held up to some crazily high-pressure ideals ...

We're still constantly told what we 'should' be: from the news, from advertising images – aspiring to an impossible ideal of what a woman should look like; glowing skin, glossy hair, symmetrical features, hot bod (the list goes on ...). Oh, and we now have social media, trolls and bullies adding their opinions on us to all of that.

We're expected to be so many things: a great partner, girlfriend, wife, friend, mother, sister, daughter, colleague, boss, change-maker, money-maker, eco warrior ... and it can be pretty damn exhausting, right?!

We're under constant pressure to upgrade our relationship status:

**When you're single it's,
'When are you getting a boyfriend/girlfriend, then?'**

**When you do have a boyfriend/girlfriend it's,
'Oh, when are they/you going to propose, then?'**

**When you're engaged it's,
'When's the wedding?'**

**When you're married it's,
'When are you having babies?'**

**When you have a baby it's,
'When are you having your second?'**

All of these questions can sound harmless to some, but for others there's so much more to it. We have our private dreams, so you never really know what the reality is, what that woman is going through. When I was younger, we didn't really think twice about quizzing our friends; we would get excited and plan our futures together. But over the past few years I've stopped asking. I've let them speak to me without prompting.

There's always going to be the 'what's next?' culture, convincing us we need to keep achieving more, more, more. Let's not add to the chase. Let's allow things to happen, without the pressure on ourselves and others.

Noise noise, noisy <u>noise</u>

Nowadays, we can't just put on fancy noise-cancelling headphones to block out all the external noise. Our phones radiate noise, and social media amplifies that noise – and Trolly McTroll faces turn that noise up so loud, SOMETIMES you feel like your ears are going to explode. We just have to sift through the wild digital noise and try to make sense of it all.

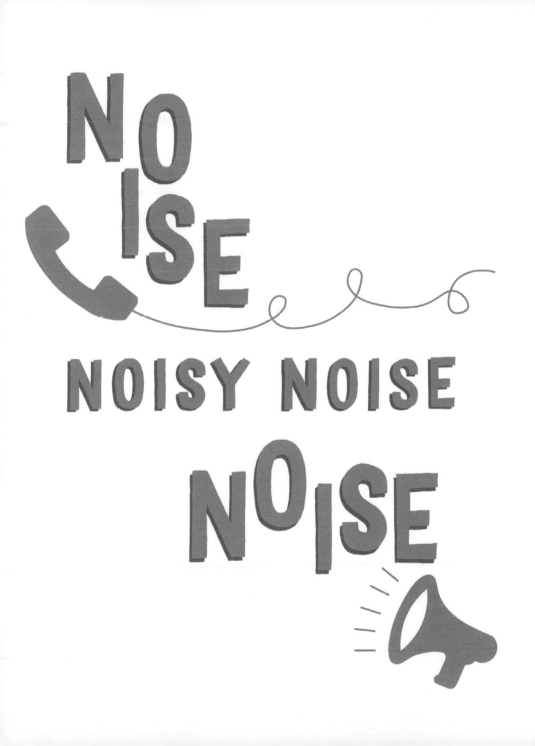

THESE ARE SOME DELIGHTFUL THINGS THAT REALLY DELIGHTFUL HUMANS HAVE SAID ABOUT ME ONLINE ...

@annonymous She's so fatty

@imabullywbu Your legs are soooo big, it's the worst

@unsolicitedadvice Large salty legs without muscles

@hidingbehindscreen And stomach that looks thick with cellulite

@bodyshamer The ideal weight for you is -10kg

@hairexpert Why moustaches for brows?

@feelingcute You're ugly, your face is still ugly

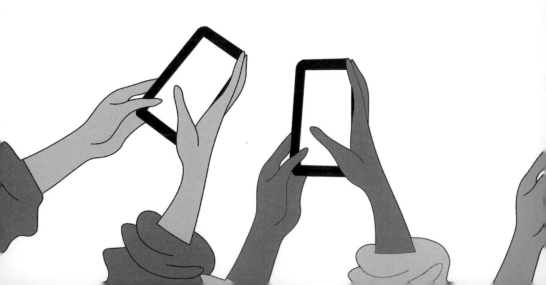

@positivity101 When you smile you have no lips

@barberboi Greasy hair, skanky roots

@trollymctrollface Her voice is so annoying

@nastayyy She's got that gross orange eye shadow on

@Keyboardwarrior She has no skill at all

@proboxer_69 The smug face she pulls makes me want
to punch it

@instabully I think you're trying to be sexy,
you look cringe and deranged

@ohpurrlease I've only been following you for
5 seconds and you're already annoying me

@animalexpert You shouldn't wear those leggings, we
can see your camel toe

@oveadig What have you done with your hair,
that colour just washes you out

90s Kiddo

Social media is everywhere now, but as I'm a 90s kid, it wasn't when I was growing up. The thrill of MSN Messenger was the closest I got to socialising online and even that wasn't until I was 11. Conversations went something a little like this ...

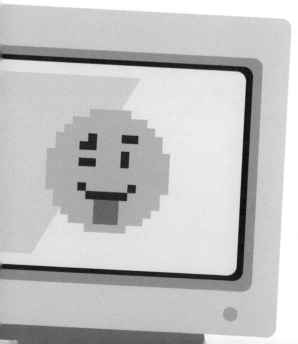

'Wubu2' [What have you been up to since I said goodbye to you at school 40 minutes ago?]

'NM, U?' [Not much because it's only been 40 minutes, you?]

'BRB' [Be right back, my mum needs to call someone on the house phone and I need to get off]

'K I G2G ANYWAY [3' [Okay, I've got to go anyway because one of the boys I fancy has just come online and he can't see I'm online at the same time because that will seem too keen ... side ice cream cone/heart]

It was our escape from school, our first discovery of the online world. My first email address was idontneedyourattitudeivegotenoughofmyown@hotmail.com. Our texts had to be within a certain number of characters otherwise you'd end up paying for two texts (15p too much!). The closest I ever got to a selfie was taken on the 0.02 megapixel webcam stuck on the top of my box of a computer. I only ever took pictures when I took my camera on my school trips, and when I came home I made photo albums from the take-your-film-to-be-developed-and-printed, blurry-AF photos. I couldn't zoom in on them to see how I looked; I just saw the whole picture, the memory captured. No filters. No editing. No Instagram. No YouTube.

There was just ... Bebo (which I only recently discovered was an acronym for blog early, blog often ... who knew?). Oh Bebo, you were revolutionary! But now I look back, you were pretty brutal. The top 16 'favourite people' on show to the world, ranked daily, based on who gave you their 'luv' (a bit similar to 'likes' on Insta but you only had three to give out a day). The 'who's hotter?' polls. The visible percentages screaming in the face of the person who lost.

But, we only spent an hour or two at most on it a day. We didn't document our lives on it, we didn't watch everyone else's lives on it. When it was Mother's Day, or our best friend's birthday, we made them a card and bought them a present. Posting a photo on Bebo with a caption saying how much we loved them wasn't cool. Posting a photo with Avril Lavigne lyrics as the captions, however, was cool.

Unsocial media

First Myspace came. Then Facebook came. Then Twitter came. Then WhatsApp came. Then Instagram came. And with all of that, came a social-media-phenomenon-fixation proven to be even more addictive than smoking and alcohol.

This planet has roughly 7.7 billion humans on it; 3.2 billion of us are active on social media daily. We are more connected than we've ever been in the history of time.

I use it. You most likely use it. The majority of people around you use it. I hear more negative press about it than positive, but that is absolutely valid. That's why I feel such a huge responsibility to use my platform and voice on social media to help as many people as I can. Especially young boys and girls growing up able to access the whole world – good and bad – in their pockets.

My newsfeed used to be a sea of perfection … and I was swimming in it. I was one of the sharks scaring people out of the water, posting silly 'perfect' pictures of me posey-posing with too much make-up and not enough honesty. No one likes swimming with sharks; they're scary, they're intimidating and you can't get close to them. I look back at old photos, posts from a few years ago, and see a different Chessie – a Chessie who cared more about looking good than doing good.

It was a classic case of monkey see, monkey do. That was Instagram back then. Inedible but stunningly curated plates of food. No squishy bits. No wobbly bits. Just everyone's best bits. So I just did what everyone else was doing: I fixated on my legs, a part of my body I fought so hard to change with diet, exercise and silly gadgets that did absolutely nothing. Everyone else's legs looked long and toned – in my eyes, the legs I wanted.

I was 21, it was new for us all, and a girl I was working with showed me an editing app she'd just paid 99p for. It was the first time I'd seen something like it. In my mini-modelling stint I'd watched photographers edit my body on photoshoots, but that was on a computer, on what looked like a high-tech piece of software. Not something that we could do. But this, this made it just so easy to change your body – on your phone – with a few thumb actions. This girl was doing it to all her photos. Stretching her legs so they looked longer, 'healing' the patches on her face she didn't like, scooping in her waist, shrinking her whole body so the photo looked slightly distorted (and in our brain-washed minds 'better' than the original).

I'm nearly 6 foot. My legs make up a lot of that height, but there I was starting to stretch myself to look even taller! The more I played around with it, the more I was contributing to society's warped view of the 'ideal woman' and the more I worried over people meeting me in real life, thinking I looked different from my photos on Instagram.

I'd sit next to girls on the Tube who were on these apps, morphing their bodies in front of me, not even trying to hide it. Even when I was doing the bikini comp (see page 142), when I was the tiniest I could possibly be, I'd want to be even smaller and it was effortless – just a few seconds on the app instead of months of hard work in the gym.

I honestly pray all editing apps get banned; they are truly toxic.

Revelation and revolution

You know when you have a loud fan on and your brain just gets used to it and you kinda forget it's even there? Then someone turns it off, and it feels so quiet. I turned off that constant hum in 2017 when I broke free from the fictitious Instagram perfection cult. It was nibbling away at my happiness and squishing the positive thoughts out of my brain. I had dedicated too many hours to trying to make my feed far more immaculate and impressive than my life actually was. The real breakthrough was after an enormous Sunday roast with the girls. It was early in the New Year, and I had already put a post up that read: 'This is the year of self-confidence … confidence in every form.' But it wasn't until 17 days later, on 19 January, that I put up my first really honest post.

It was nothing spectacular, just a photo of me sitting on the floor, with my flies undone and my belly poking out. As soon as I posted it, I plugged my phone in and left it in the kitchen, mainly so I wouldn't end up regretting and deleting it. It's funny, because I remember feeling so liberated but, equally, pooing my pants not knowing what the response was going to be. I woke up the next morning and the post was flooded with comments from people – 'Thank you' and 'Finally, someone I can actually relate to!' And that was just the start. I had gone from a shark to a wave in the sea.

I wanted to take everyone with me. I wanted to make a change. I thought, 'If I'm going to use social media at all, I'm going to use it to help.' The more messages I received, the more I wanted to share, the more I wanted to help pull others out of the trap, the more I wanted to scream: 'We need to stop this bullshit because it is damaging people's view of themselves and it is warping our views of our bodies.'

Obviously it wasn't all la-dee-da scrummyscrumptious. My first experience of trolling was delightful. Someone set up an anonymous account and used it to post photos of me – they put my original posts next to their Photoshopped versions (where I had been shrunk to half my size). The captions under the edited photos read: '@chessieking – better minus 10kgs'. It's ironic now I look back … I'd been doing that to myself, editing my body to make myself look smaller, but when someone did it to me, it felt like a punch in the boobies.

I was angry, really angry, and had an urge to post something to retaliate. This person was clearly so heavily invested in my life, had all the spare time to edit my body and was fixated on my every post … So, on 19 March 2017, I gave them what they wanted: I posted my first 'jiggle wiggly wibbly wobbly in my teeny weenie pants' video – 20 per cent for the troll; 80 per cent for the people that I thought needed to see it. The caption was:

So I've never posted a video exposing so much of my body and it's pretty scary (/petrifying) but I really want to share with you the bits you don't even see … We should all be allowed the body confidence we all admire. Confidence doesn't mean arrogance, it comes from a place that has developed over years and years of learning about your body. We are surrounded by modern day's perception of how we 'should' look … If we all looked the way society tells us how to look, we'd all be so similar and this would be one boring world of humans. So this week, when you're in your bedroom, living room, shower, wiggle 'n' jiggle that body of yours. If we all do it together, we might create an earthquake.

I was still working out daily at the time, I was much smaller than I am currently, but it erupted something in me and disrupted people's feeds. My message started shifting. My mission started changing.

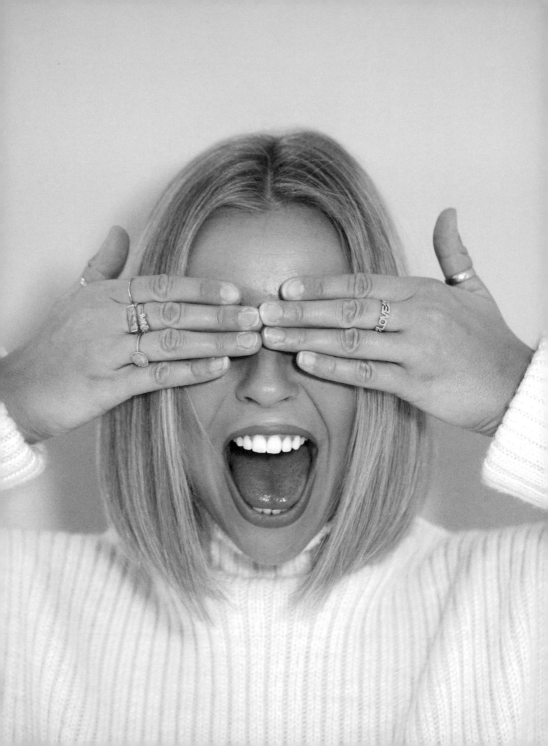

Trolly McTroll faces

The more my audience grew, the more I shared my body, the more opinions I attracted, and as a result – the more hate I got (and still get!).

At school, the boys would empty out the contents of my bag when I walked into the corridor before the start-of-lesson bell. Online, the trolls and cyberbullies would empty out the contents of my confidence tank. At school, my parents received an unsigned handwritten hate letter. Online, I've had countless death threats from faceless accounts.

There have been days when these bullies have robbed me of my voice, my happiness and my time. But with experience and as I've grown up, I've realised it's not about me. It's nothing to do with me. It's them. Unhappy, malicious, sad, sad people. I genuinely wish the best for them and hope they find a way out of such a dark place. There have been countless times when I've been so close to coming off social media and deleting my Instagram account to escape it all.

I've worked with cyberbullying charities to create awareness through powerful campaigns, but most importantly, to help anyone who's been affected by bullying. I have witnessed the damage it can do and the extreme places it can take victims to. It happens to people with 23 followers or 2.3 million followers. I've discovered that trolls all rally together on forums. They'll create a plan of attack and try to annihilate a post together with their revolting comments – it's like they thrive off doing it with others. It's going back to that feeling of community, feeling a part of something, but they're using their voices for absolutely the wrong reasons.

My mission to help victims of trolling and cyberbullying is to do everything I can to be the voice that they need to hear. We can get through it together and they will not win.

MY TOP TIPS ON HOW TO DEAL WITH BULLYING

★ Tell someone in your solar support system. Don't just keep it to yourself – try to read the comment out loud in a silly voice, make a face, shout it out and take away its power.

★ Block the account and delete the comment. Out of sight. Out of mind.

★ Get help and professional support if it continues. Do not suffer in solitude – there is an army of help out there.

★ If you see anyone or know anyone getting targeted online, don't feed the troll. As much as you want to stick up for them in the comments section, you're giving the trolls what they want –attention. Instead, privately message the person being targeted and recommend the above. Show your support, show them they're not battling alone. Listen to them. Understand how much it's affecting them.

★ Give your comments some thought. The phrase used to be 'Think before you speak' but now it's a case of 'Think before you comment'. Don't use your thumbs as weapons.

★ I find repeating what these strangers say about me so liberating. It's actually where my one and only theme tune – 'I don't care what you think of me' – came from. I try to impersonate the haters and their comments in ridiculous accents/characters with silly faces either to myself or I put on a show for Mat! By doing it, I feel like I'm taking back control, like I'm in charge of how these people make me feel.

★ If you have been told by family and friends 'you're so negative', 'just get over it', or 'you're a massive burden' then there are some phenomenal charities who are just a phone call away – I promise you are not alone and they'll make you feel heard: Cybersmile, Samaritans, Maytree and Give Us a Shout.

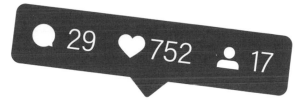

WINstagram

Social media can be a source of inspiration, joy and entertainment – as much as it can be something that grabs and twists your nips, making you want to scream.

I've really learnt how to make sure we're using it for good, but more importantly, to make us feel good. A year ago, I set out to use my voice on social media to try to change the school curriculum. I've been campaigning for an hour a week (at least) to cover body confidence, mental-health awareness, social-media usage and all the shit I wish I'd been taught. I want to make a stand for our younger brothers and sisters, our future generation and our teachers who need the extra support more than ever. I feel I can bridge the gap between parents and their children, and act as a middle ground for teachers and students. We are being heard, by the Department of Education in the UK, which is incredible. It's something I am extremely dedicated to – which is why I called it 'Dedicate to Educate'.

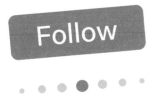

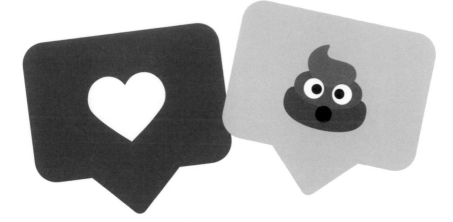

Is your Instagram a WINstagram or a shit-stagram...?

Be honest with yourself and answer a few questions on how you use social media. It might just help you clean up your feed.

1. IS IT A PLACE WHERE YOU CONNECT WITH PEOPLE/COMMUNITIES AND LEAVE FEELING EMPOWERED?

A. Yes   B. No   C. Sometimes

(If yes or sometimes, write down the last time you felt like this)

2. IS IT A PLACE WHERE YOU GO TO FEEL INSPIRED?

A. Yes   B. No   C. Sometimes

(If yes or sometimes, write down the last time you felt like this)

3. IS IT AN ESCAPE FROM REAL LIFE?

A. Yes   B. No   C. Sometimes

(If yes or sometimes, write down the last time you felt like this)

4. IS IT A PLACE YOU GO TO SCROLL WHEN YOU'RE FEELING WEAK AND SELF-DESTRUCTIVE, AND THEN IT ENDS UP MAKING YOU FEEL EVEN WORSE?

A. Yes   B. No   C. Sometimes

(if yes or sometimes, go back to your list of things that make you happy from page 67 and do one of these when you next reach for your phone.)

What's your feed feeding you?

Inspiring stories.

Diet culture.

Puppies.

Waist trainers.

Diversity.

People putting down other people.

Art.

Advice from trained nutritionists.

Unsolicited advice.

Your friends doing things without you.

Talent.

Educational captions.

People who
are using their
platforms for good.

Photographs
of nature.

FAKE NEWS.

Unrealistic and
unattainable
workouts.

Relatable and
easy-to-follow
yoga videos.

Babies.

Edited/photoshopped
bodies.

People eating
four grapes
for breakfast.

People's lives
that open you
up to different
viewpoints.

Positive
affirmations.

How many oranges have you selected?
How many reds have you chosen?

If you've picked more than two reds, you need to unfollow, mute,
block and get rid of those accounts that are clogging up your feed
with their bullshit.

Unpack your suitcase

You know when you're at the airport check-in and the person asks you, 'Has anyone packed your bags for you?' while pointing at a sheet listing dangerous goods? I don't think I've ever said anything other than no – have you? Well, that's one way to look at your Instagram. You would never let anyone pack your suitcase with weapons, would you? So why would you let people fill your Insta feed with damaging shit that's going to make you feel like shit? If you're packing your case with heavy reds, we need to offload them – they're weighing you down, you've gone way over the baggage allowance! So unfollow, mute, do whatever you need to do. Take personal responsibility.

THINGS I'VE LEARNT ABOUT INSTAGRAM

★ **To accept that images won't be 100 per cent 'real'** and people will still post doctored/posed/staged photos. I follow some of these accounts for their beautiful photography – to me, it's a form of art and I look at it with that mindset. It's a reflection of their creativity and a platform to show different talents. I don't follow anyone who photoshops their body or face, just the environment/background.

★ **The loudest voices aren't always the right voices.** I don't value someone's advice any more if they have a bigger audience. Some medical professionals with extremely informative and educational posts sharing their knowledge on social media only have a few thousand followers, but they can be overshadowed by unqualified advice from bigger platforms. It's hard to know what's right, but just remind yourself: big following doesn't equal big brains.

★ **Don't use it as a place to tear people down.** I have never and will never use Instagram to speak negatively about a person, a brand or a company. I see so many people doing it and airing their injustice to the world, but I honestly find that one of the most negative sides of the online world. I will send someone an email or a direct message if I feel let down by them or if they've done something to upset me; I would never take to publicly shaming them or shouting them out.

★ **Public means public.** I used to think my profile was a 'safe space' for us all, but it's not. If you have a public account, it's open to the **public,** so trolls have access just like the rest of us. Sometimes online bullies will not just comment on **me** and my photos, but also reply to my follower's comments, and I have to be on the lookout for that to protect them.

★ **Phones are the most distracting thing in the entire universe.** They can literally take your attention away from any situation. Even when I'm out for dinner and I've turned the screen down flat on the table, I'll be tempted to turn it over to google how long it took a man to roll a Brussels sprout up a mountain with his nose ... next thing we'll be engrossed in a 25-minute YouTube video ... and by that time your food's cold, you've looked at the Brussels sprout more than you have the person you're out for dinner with. Just put it in your bag or somewhere you can't easily grab it.

★ **No one cares if your Instagram Stories aren't going up instantly.** When you're out with friends and family, trying to perfect your stories like you're some kinda Van Gogh is not the best use of your time ... trust me. Take photos/videos throughout the day and post them as a round-up later. They don't need to be live; no one's going to cry if you post your brunch pancakes at 5pm. You don't want to look back at all the times you went out for breakfast with your mum but spent the entire time trying to find the funniest food GIF.

YOU CONTROL YOUR PHONE, DON'T LET IT CONTROL YOU

★ Turn off all notifications. Even the '50 per cent off all clothes, buy now or regret later' on your favourite clothes app. Your brain does not need the constant ping-ping-ping-ing.

★ Make your bedroom a phone-free zone. Mat and I leave ours in the living room.

★ Put on your favourite podcast and then put your phone away in your bag (backpacks are the best so it's not as easy to reach in and get it) until it finishes.

★ Reply back to your friends/family before you reply to a comment/direct message from a stranger/follower.

★ Swap your lunchtime scroll and go get your daily dose of nature. Take yourself outside for a little walk or lock yourself in a bathroom cubicle and do a little wiggle.

★ Have a notebook to take into bed with you. Every evening I write down five things I need to do the next day for work and five things I want to do for myself.

★ Scroll-free Sundays are a dream. I reply back to a few messages in the morning, then leave my phone until 6 p.m.-ish. It's just a mini-insight into a tech-free life and it's so refreshing.

★ Try 10 minutes of tech-free stillness every day – if 10 minutes sounds too much, start off with two minutes of just sitting in silence, then add on two minutes every week.

★ Just breathe … in for four, hold for four, out for four, hold for four. Repeat. Do it now.

YOU CONTROL YOUR PHONE

DON'T LET IT CONTROL YOU

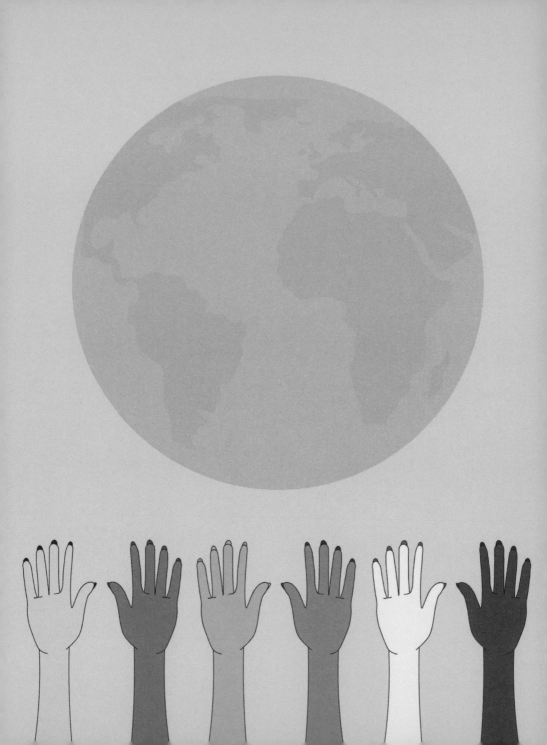

Connecting with women all around the world

Not long ago, I was flying home from a wedding in Greece with Mat. We sat down in our row, next to a lady already in the window seat. As soon as I'd buckled myself in and stopped stuffing the pocket in front of me with all our snacks, I noticed her legs bouncing up and down and, paired with her audible breath, I'm not embarrassed to admit that my first thought was that she was drunk.

As we were lining ourselves up on the runway ready to take off, her breath became more panicky and her whole chair started gyrating. I realised that in fact she was having a panic attack and was most likely absolutely terrified of flying. I felt her fear inside me and immediately wanted to help her. As the plane gathered speed, I put my hand on her leg, she put her hand on top of mine and squeezed it tight. We sat in silence holding hands, as strangers, connected through touch and understanding.

She turned to me with tears rolling down her face when we were finally floating up in the clouds. She thanked me again and again and said I had calmed her down more than I knew. She told me she had three children and one of them had panic attacks every time they went on a plane and so she had also developed a phobia of flying. She apologised for being silly as she was a grown woman, but I assured her I was a professional calmer-downer after years of holding Brontë's hand on every take-off we've ever done together!

Now, I'm not saying you need to go and hold strangers' hands, or even touch anyone you don't know … I don't want anyone getting reported for grabbing anonymous hands! I'm also not being that person who buys a sandwich for a homeless person, then posts it all over their social media to prove they've done it. I'm not looking for applause. I'm just reiterating that everyone has their own story and, as women, we can be kind and empathetic towards other women. We can all take a little extra time to recognise our similarities.

The woman who's juggling a screaming baby and a truck-of-a-pram on the bus is probably screaming inside herself – with embarrassment. Instead of huffing and puffing and wishing the kid would **shut up**, go and ask if you can help them. That would be lovely, wouldn't it!

When I was 18 I trained to be a massage therapist under the wing of an incredible integrated health doctor, Dr A. I worked in his clinic in London and later went on to be a live-in therapist for a month in Oman, specialising in stroke patients and anyone coming out of a neck- or back-related injury. Dr A looked after a handful of families where their religion didn't allow the women to be massaged by him. So, when I was all trained up, he passed those clients on to me. They would walk in the room on their first visit a stranger, but even after just an hour together, they would leave a friend. I heard stories that are unspeakable and it gave me even more of an awareness of how women are treated in different cultures and what they go through.

I think it's incredibly important to surround yourself with diversity, to understand and learn about other women's lives. Inject a little extra love into the world today and offer a hand, not just to women, to anyone.

'IF ONLY OUR EYES SAW THROUGH TO PEOPLE'S SOULS INSTEAD OF THEIR BODIES, HOW VERY DIFFERENT THE IDEAL OF BEAUTY WOULD BE...'

You VS the outer orbit

Throughout the different chapters of your book there are going to be a handful of strangers who will always make assumptions about you before they know you. Online, they'll form their opinion of you based on the first six squares on your Instagram page. Offline, they'll judge you for the book you're reading on the train or what you're wearing at a wedding.

But you know yourself better than anyone, and that's the magic trick – as long as you know who you are, what you like, what makes you happy, then who gives a fuck what anyone else sees?

'Other peoples' opinions of you is none of your business.'

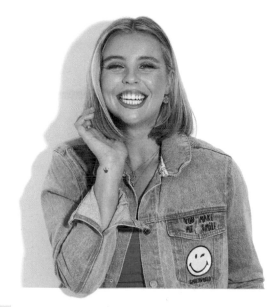

Be the same
person
privately,
publicly
and personally.
Don't change
yourself for
anyone.

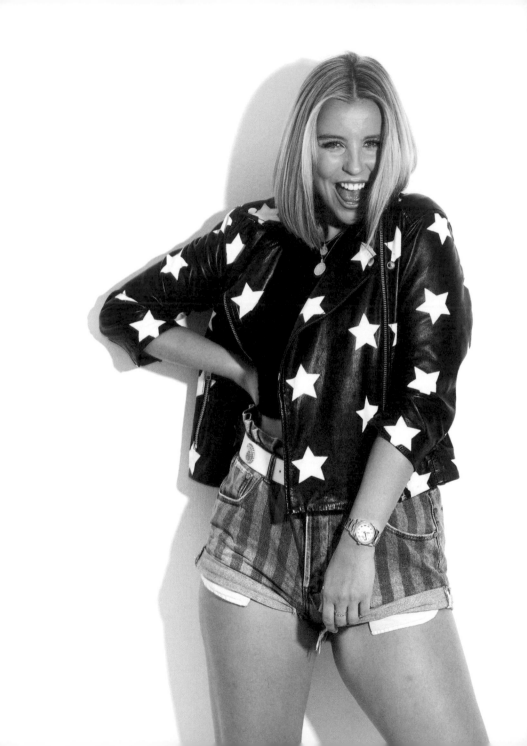

Hopefully, throughout this book you've strengthened your relationship with yourself, your best friend. The more you believe in yourself and know your true worth and value, the less you're going to care what strangers think of you.

I hope it's also made you empathise with other women and what we're all going through daily. We need to unwrap ourselves, take ourselves out of our own universe and open our eyes to what's going on in other people's inner worlds. We never know what anyone else has been through or is going through. Being a compassionate and kind human being is much, much more valuable than having a hot bod. Stand up for yourself and for each other. Bring people up. Be a radiator, but keep some of that warmth for you and your best friend. Infect people with your contagious energy.

Here's a big dollop of thank you, topped with one huge gigantic enormous handful of love sprinkled on top of that appreciation. You made it to the end (or you've just skipped to the back like I do with most of my books when I want to know what happens!). We did it together. I genuinely have tears rolling down my face right now, but I am elated for both of us. I wish I had my arms wrapped around you, squeezing you – I feel so connected to you knowing you've read through until this last page.

I really do adore you and I'm sending you an endless amount of self-belief my sister, friend, reader.

I really do adore you,

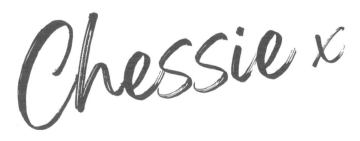

Thank yous

IT'S THE PAGE THAT ONLY THE PEOPLE WHO I THANK WILL READ...

So I want to start off the never-ending list with saying a ginormous shout out to the wonderful team at HarperCollins – the energy you all put into every meeting and the freedom you gave me to create all 240 pages.

Thank you to Becky for filtering through and making sense of the jumble of words we started with. You helped shape the book, teased out the spicy details and guided me with your experience.

A super special thank you to Saskia – my extremely talented illustrator, who jumps inside my chaotic brain and creates something pretty magic out of my messy scribbles.

The faaaaabulous Ruth Rose for being so talented and being my hype girl when I took all my clothes off for the nuuudey ruuudey shots!

Mr Andrew Selby (page 196's Doris minus the boobies) – an absolute champion who surpasses the 'manager' role with his unlimited supply of support.

Mathew sensational Carter – thank you for believing in me, thank you for searching through your built-in personal dictionary for synonyms when I'd used 'phenomenal' too many times and for asking me to be your wife ... Mrs King Carter.

Thank you Mumma, Daddadio, Bee and H for giving me the level of love that makes me feel invincible.

My Twin, Niige, Angel Skye, G, Hels, Jenners, Babybird, Hazelnut, Vera, Ernie, Alice, Rhi Rhi, Toriebird, Lozza & Annabib. Really truuuuly adore you forever + ever.

AND A HUUUUGE DOLLOP OF APPRECIATION FOR YOU x